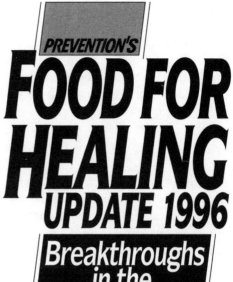

PREVENTION'S FOOD FOR HEALING UPDATE 1996

Breakthroughs in the Curative Power of Nutrition

Edited by
Mark Bricklin, Editor,
PREVENTION Magazine,
and Julia Hansen,
PREVENTION Magazine
Health Books

Rodale Press, Inc.
Emmaus, Pennsylvania

Copyright © 1996 by Rodale Press, Inc.

Printed in the United States of America on acid-free (∞), recycled paper ♻

ISBN 0–87596–303–X   hardcover

Distributed in the book trade by St. Martin's Press

2   4   6   8   10   9   7   5   3   1   hardcover

OUR MISSION
We publish books that empower people's lives.

RODALE BOOKS

Prevention's Food for Healing Update 1996 **Editorial Staff**

Editor: **Julia Hansen**
Managing Editor: **Sharon Faelten**
Permissions Coordinator: **Anita Small**
Fact-Checker: **Carol J. Gilmore**
Copy Editor: **Kathy Diehl**
Cover Designer: **Richard Rossiter**
Book Designer: **Kristen Morgan Downey**
Associate Art Director: **Faith Hague**
Studio Manager: **Joe Golden**
Technical Artist: **David Q. Pryor**
Page Layout: **Sharon M. Seng**
Office Staff: **Roberta Mulliner, Julie Kehs,**
          Bernadette Sauerwine, Mary Lou Stephen
Production Manager: **Helen Clogston**
Manufacturing Coordinator: **Melinda B. Rizzo**

Rodale Health and Fitness Books

Vice-President and Editorial Director: **Debora T. Yost**
Art Director: **Jane Colby Knutila**
Research Manager: **Ann Gossy Yermish**
Copy Manager: **Lisa D. Andruscavage**

Contents

Part I
Nutrition News: This Just In

The latest medical reports on the ever-strengthening link
between diet and good health.

Part II
Foods for Better Health

....

Your diet can have a powerful effect on how you feel—and heal. Here's what (and how) to eat to help prevent disease, relieve symptoms, speed recovery, shed extra pounds and generally heal what ails you.

Part III
Healing with Vitamins: The Year's Breakthroughs

Researchers and doctors are studying the potential healing properties of vitamins as never before, and the news is encouraging. Here's how to power up your own diet.

Vitamins and Beyond

Part IV
Prevention Cuisine: Low-Fat at Its Best

Eating healthfully doesn't mean you can't eat well. These recipes, cooking tips and shopping hints can help keep you nutritionally fit for life.

Introduction
Your Eat-to-Heal Action Plan

WE AT *PREVENTION* KNEW it all the time. Now the news shouts from every morning talk show and evening newscast: What we eat—or don't eat—can and does affect our health.

It would be easy to laugh at such an obvious truth, if the truth weren't so confusing. We all know that a banana is a healthier snack than a sticky bun. But trying to navigate the blizzard of often contradictory nutritional information has left many of us throwing up our hands in bewilderment.

Should we swallow vitamin supplements or get our vitamins through food? Is it true that margarine is just as bad as butter? Will following a vegetarian diet improve your health or deprive your body of crucial nutrients? And perhaps most important: How come you're eating low-fat everything but still gaining weight?

Exit nutritional confusion. Enter *Prevention's Food for Healing Update 1996.*

This book presents the cutting edge of nutritional research *plus* specific eat-to-heal strategies created by doctors to help you treat or prevent disease, lose weight and keep it off, uplift your mood, ease pain and more. Here are just a few of the nutritional breakthroughs you'll find in these pages.

- Soy foods like tofu contain compounds found to help ease the hot flashes associated with menopause and may even thwart breast cancer.
- Evidence reveals that eating more often can help you shed pounds. What's more, indulging an occasional yen for chocolate or chips may be smarter than trying to white-knuckle it through a craving.

- Scientific research has linked depression to a deficiency of B vitamins in some people.
- Many people with arthritis who follow a vegetarian diet experience dramatic relief from stiff, painful joints.

You'll find the book simple to use, too. Part 1, "Nutrition News," presents still-unfolding breakthroughs in nutrition research. Part 2, "Foods for Better Health," is packed with food "prescriptions" that can help prevent or treat a variety of health conditions, from arthritis to osteoporosis. Part 3, "Healing with Vitamins," reveals how certain nutrients may short-circuit heart trouble, sharpen your memory and deflate high blood pressure.

But food is more than mere fuel: It should tantalize the taste buds and soothe the soul, too. So part 4, "*Prevention* Cuisine," features a collection of mouth-watering, no-guilt treats. You'll feast on lasagna, Mexican food and other formerly forbidden dishes while you enjoy optimum health.

The goal of this book? To help you view every meal as an opportunity to give yourself the gift of a longer, healthier life. And to show you how rewarding taking control of your health can be.

We at *Prevention* always knew that, too.

Mark Bricklin
Prevention Magazine

Part I

Nutrition News: This Just In

"Island Diet" Promotes Heart Health

THE ISLAND OF CRETE is not just on the Mediterranean Sea; it's in it. No wonder then that the people of that island lying off the coast of Greece enjoy what's called Mediterranean cuisine—tasty fare with little meat or rich foods but large amounts of vegetables, fruits, grains and fish along with fairly generous splashes of both olive oil and wine.

The people of Crete also enjoy an astonishingly low rate of heart disease. One scientific project, called the Seven Countries Study, found that while 46 percent of deaths among middle-aged American men were a result of heart disease, that number in Crete was a mere 4 percent—ten times less. In fact, the death rate for any and all causes in Crete during the 15-year study was lower than in any other country studied. Why?

Probing the Diet Link

Researchers in France decided to find out. Some years ago, medical researchers began working with about 600 men, each of whom had had a recent heart attack. Half the group was told to eat the "prudent" low-fat diet prescribed in many nations. The other half was told to follow a "Mediterranean diet" that strongly resembled the Cretan diet.

Here are the specific instructions that the Mediterranean-diet group received during dietary counseling.

1. Eat more vegetables of all kinds.
2. Eat more fruit of any kind—"no day without fruit."
3. Eat more bread.
4. Eat more fish.

2

5. Lay off meat; eat it no more than once a day and replace beef, lamb and pork with poultry.
6. No butter, cream or milk.
7. Drink moderate amounts of wine with meals, if desired.
8. For salads and cooking, use olive oil or canola oil exclusively.

Just how well did this diet perform, versus the "standard" diet given to most heart patients?

Spectacularly well. In the group of patients following the Mediterranean diet, there were nearly 70 percent fewer heart attacks and subsequent cardiac deaths. The benefits kicked in early, too—in just a matter of months.

Supreme Eating

What's also important is that these people were eating a diet not just featuring olive or canola oil in place of butter or other fats but a diet that was low overall in saturated fats as well. That's the kind of fat that's truly terrible for your ticker and found mostly in butter, cream and fatty meats.

The fact is, it's possible that the reduction in saturated fats alone was largely responsible for the apparently good results, according to Margo Denke, M.D., associate professor of medicine at the University of Texas Southwestern Medical Center for Human Nutrition at Dallas. Dr. Denke also believes that if the group getting the "standard" low-fat diet had been given counseling on how to eat the low saturated fat diet like the other group received, they might have done much better.

Perhaps that is true. Certainly, we have to say now that the best dietary change you can make is to steer clear of those saturated fats mentioned above.

What really needs to be done is for the Mediterranean diet to be tried in a country that's nowhere near the Mediterranean, such as the United States or England, says Serge Renaud, Ph.D., of France's National Institute of Health and Medical Research. Then we'd see if the "magic" of the Mediterranean is a universal law or just another island dream.

....

Olive Oil Boosts "Good" Cholesterol

OLIVE OIL MAY BE THE modern genie in a bottle, driving out the artery-clogging type of cholesterol (low-density lipoprotein, or LDL) without diminishing the helpful kind (high-density lipoprotein, or HDL). Now researchers are beginning to find out how it works its magic. A recent French study suggests that the monounsaturated fat in the oil may actually change the chemical composition of HDL, making it more efficient in rousting LDL.

Researchers tested lipid levels of 12 women who were placed on four different seven-week diets, all with 30 percent of total calories derived from fat. The largest portion of fat in each group came from a different source: either milk fats (saturated fat), sunflower oil (high in omega-6 polyunsaturates), rapeseed oil (canola oil; high in omega-3 polyunsaturates) or olive oil (high in monounsaturates).

With the olive oil diet, researchers not only saw the greatest drop in LDL, they also saw HDL become smaller and more fluid, which may help it remove cholesterol from cells more effectively. The other diets, though, actually made the HDL less fluid.

"This finding helps explain how higher HDL levels may protect against heart disease and how monounsaturated fats might play a helpful role; however, more research is needed," says lipid expert Margo Denke, M.D., associate professor of medicine at the University of Texas Southwestern Medical Center for Human Nutrition at Dallas.

Now this doesn't mean you should start spooning olive oil over everything. As you may already know, *Prevention* magazine's rule is to keep calories from fat below 25 percent of the day's total calorie intake. You can make a few constructive switches, however, if you think Mediterranean: Try substituting olive oil for your usual cooking oil or use its subtle taste in place of butter on bread.

Give Trans Fats the Slip

THE BATTLE RAGES ON to decide which slippery character is worse for blood cholesterol levels—the saturated fat found in butter, cheese, whole milk, ice cream and meat or the trans-fatty acids used in margarines, commercially baked goods and french fries.

Trans-Form Your Diet

It's estimated that Americans consume 8 to 13 grams of trans-fatty acids daily. Here's the trans-fatty acid content of restaurant and store-bought foods analyzed at Harvard University.

FOOD	TRANS-FATTY ACIDS (g.)
4 ounces fast-food french fries	3.43
1 danish pastry	3.03
1 ounce corn chips	1.42
1 piece cake	1.04
1 piece pie	1.00
1 cookie	0.86
1 teaspoon vegetable shortening	0.63
1 teaspoon stick margarine	0.62
1 teaspoon tub margarine	0.27
1 teaspoon vegetable oil	0.02
1 teaspoon reduced-calorie mayonnaise	0.01

The American Heart Association and top associations of nutrition scientists say that research shows the worst offender by far is the saturated fat (and cholesterol) in butter. But two scientists at the Harvard School of Public Health made news by tagging trans-fatty acids (created when food processors add hydrogen to vegetable oil) as the nastier of the two.

The main point is that there's evidence that too much of either fat helps choke arteries with plaque.

Currently, food processors aren't required to reveal the amount of trans-fatty acids they add to products, so there's no way to know exactly how much is hidden in food you buy. But check out the ingredients list. If any partially hydrogenated vegetable oil is listed in the first few ingredients—especially in a food high in total fat—chances are there's more than a trickle of trans-fatty acids.

Want to give the slip to high levels of trans-fatty acids? You can. Simply follow these tips and trim your intake of trans fats.

- Eat a healthy low-fat diet. Food that's low in fat will automatically be low in both trans-fatty acids and saturated fat.
- If you can't do without a bread spread, choose reduced-fat or fat-free margarine over butter or stick margarine.
- For sautéing choose fat-free liquids, cooking sprays or small amounts of vegetable oil or liquid margarine.
- Look for low-fat commercially baked goods, especially ones that are made with vegetable oils that haven't been partially hydrogenated.
- Put french fries, pastries and chips in the once-in-a-while-only contingent.

Going Green May Save Your Sight

GREEN MAY BE THE NEXT great color for eyes. Leafy verdant vegetables such as spinach and collard greens could protect your peepers against the leading cause of blindness in people over age 65.

So far, diet looks like the only promising way to thwart the onset of this disease, called macular degeneration. The advanced form strikes about 1 in 100 people by age 65. By age 75 the risk is 1 in 20.

Earlier studies hinted that nutrients called antioxidants could stave off this disease, in which blood vessels in the macula (part of the retina) develop sight-blocking leaks. This study provides the first evidence regarding diet: People who consumed the highest amounts of carotenoids lowered their risk of macular degeneration by 43 percent compared with people who ate the least. This study also suggests that two specific carotenoids—lutein and zeaxanthin—are most strongly associated with a reduction in risk. With regard to specific foods, eating a half-cup of spinach or collard greens per week or more often was associated with a lower risk, and the more often the better.

Those exotic-sounding nutrients aren't hard to find: This study pinpointed spinach and collard greens as offering the most benefits, but the nutrients are also plentiful in kale, mustard greens, turnip greens, parsley and dill. Lutein and zeaxanthin are present but a little more sparse in broccoli, brussels sprouts, raw leeks, leaf lettuce, celery, squash and pumpkin. Researchers discerned this reduction in risk after polling 356 people with macular degeneration and 520 without on their eating habits.

Since the macula contains polyunsaturated fatty acids, it may be particularly susceptible to damage from the free radicals created in the course of simply living through a day. (Free radicals are unstable molecules that damage cells and tissues.) The two carotenoids mentioned may disarm those radicals enough to leave the cells—and your sight—in good working order, says Johanna M. Seddon, M.D., associate professor of ophthalmology and epidemiology at Harvard Medical School and Harvard School of Public Health.

"The study showed that more frequent intake of these nutrients and foods was better," she says. "The maximum reduction in risk was 80 percent for people who consumed these vegetables five or more times per week, though there were few people in this category, so we have to be cautious."

So should you start to holler for collards? "It seems prudent," says Dr. Seddon, to eat more vegetables, particularly dark green, leafy ones, which are high in these particular carotenoids. Even if you've never handled them before, collards, kale or other greens can be turned into tasty dishes without a whole lot of research. Dice these greens and place them where you'd use broccoli on a pizza. Or make a 60-second side dish by sautéing these greens with a little olive oil. Get creative with spices: Try ginger, cardamom, cinnamon, nutmeg, ginger, chili pepper or garlic.

Salad-Bar Garnish a Nutritional Gold Mine

THE NUTRITIONAL SUPERSTAR of the salad bar may be a great-looking veggie that we're not intended to eat. It's kale—those ruffly, dark green leaves tucked around the salad-ingredient crocks for decoration only and then tossed away by the ton.

But look what we're wasting: Kale has four times as much beta-carotene as broccoli, and a half-cup contains as much vitamin C as half an orange. Plus kale is bursting with other intriguing compounds that scientists think may help ward off cancer and heart disease. It's the highest known source of lutein, a carotenoid linked to lower rates of lung cancer. It's among the highest known sources of antioxidant flavonoids, which are linked to lower rates of fatal heart attack. And it's a source of two substances now being studied as breast cancer fighters—sulforaphane and indole-3-carbinol. Try kale steamed and seasoned with caraway or fennel seeds, stir-fried with lean pork, ginger and garlic or in soups with beans, barley and potatoes.

Tomatoes Soup Up Cancer Protection

CAN A *TOMATO* A DAY keep the doctor away? Maybe. Scientists found recently that people in northern Italy who ate seven or more servings of raw tomatoes a week had 60 percent less chance of developing colon, rectal and stomach cancer than people who ate two servings or less. In fact, eating tomatoes was linked to even less risk of cancer than eating fruits or green vegetables. And a decade ago, Harvard Medical School researcher Graham Colditz, M.D., found that older Americans who often ate tomatoes were only half as likely to die from all cancers combined.

What's so plummy about tomatoes? According to Dr. Colditz, tomatoes are one of the few foods rich in an antioxidant called lycopene, a member of the carotenoid clan, that's been overshadowed till now by its famous cousin, beta-carotene. Scientists think that antioxidants from veggies and fruits become commandos against cancer inside our bodies.

(Besides lycopene, tomatoes have vitamin C and p-courmaric and cholorgenic acids—even *more* antioxidants!)

Luckily, lycopene survives heating. That means you'll find it in processed tomato products. So if eating plain tomatoes every day sounds pretty monotonous, think angel-hair pasta with tomato sauce instead. Or three-bean chili. Or vegetable juice cocktail. The other top sources? Watermelon, pink grapefruit and guava.

Spoon Up Cranberries, Stave Off Aging

THINGS WE LOVE ABOUT cranberry sauce: first, the tart, sweet flavor. Second, the familiar "plop" as it emerges from the can. And now, the polyphenols—antioxidant compounds found in many fruits, including cranberries. Researchers who extracted polyphenols from cranberries found them to be efficient scavengers of troublesome free radicals—unstable molecules that can wreak havoc on cells and tissues. Free radicals may be formed by natural processes in the the body or by environmental influences such as cigarette smoke, sunlight or pollution. Antioxidants neutralize these free radicals. That may make cranberries one more delicious shield against the ills that free radicals help cause: heart disease, cancer and the deteriorating effects of aging.

Supplements May Squelch Cervical Cancer

EVERY YEAR MILLIONS OF American women learn that a routine Pap test has uncovered cervical dysplasia—telltale changes in cells of the uterus that *sometimes* lead to cervical cancer. To head off cervical dysplasia, regular checkups are vital. Your doctor may remove the suspicious cells or treat them with a laser. But an additional weapon is currently under study: beta-carotene supplements.

In preliminary tests at the University of California, Irvine, women with cervical dysplasia were given 30 milligrams of beta-carotene supplements daily for 19 months. That equals 50,000 international units a day. Six months after stopping the beta-carotene, 21 of the 30 women were free of dysplasia. Results were so promising that a much larger randomized trial now is under way. Don't try this at home, though: Check with your doctor before taking beta-carotene supplements.

Carrots, Cantaloupe KO Coronaries

CRAVING A SWEET, JUICY PEACH? A slice of fresh, fragrant cantaloupe? A steamy sweet potato? Go ahead—eat a bumper crop. These foods, along with certain other fruits and veggies, may slash your risk of a heart attack, according to a recent study.

In this study researchers found that nonsmoking men who had high levels of carotenoids in their blood had 72 percent fewer heart attacks than men with the lowest levels of these compounds. Carotenoids are antioxidants and help prevent the damage to "bad" LDL cholesterol that is believed to make it stick to your arteries.

Benefits were less for the smokers in this group of 1,883 men (ages 40 to 59 when the study began). But even smokers with high levels of carotenoids still had about 25 percent fewer heart attacks in the 13 years they were studied than did men whose blood showed the lowest amounts.

Carotenoids occur naturally in fruits and vegetables, especially orange ones such as carrots, sweet potatoes, apricots, cantaloupe and peaches. There's a green team of carotenoid sources, too, including spinach, kale, collard greens and loose-leaf lettuce.

While beta-carotene is the most well-known carotenoid, "other carotenoids also have antioxidant effects," says study co-author Dexter L. Morris, M.D., Ph.D., vice-chairman of the Department of Emergency Medicine at the University of North Carolina at Chapel Hill School of Medicine.

What's more, these other carotenoids may have a larger role in good health than previously thought. "Studies are beginning to accumulate to suggest that diets that contain at least some carotenoids are probably going to be beneficial against heart disease, cancer and possibly other diseases," says Dr. Morris. "The fact that there was this much difference in risk in this study suggests there's something fairly important going on."

Dr. Morris's recommendation? Eat the produce you prefer. "While some foods contain more carotenoids than others, I'd recommend choosing vegetables that you like and that you'll be able to eat on a regular basis," he says.

Zap Diabetes with Salmon, Sardines

. THERE MAY BE EVEN MORE you can do to deter diabetes than control your weight and work your body. Recent research hints that adding fatty fish such as salmon or sardines to your diet may help keep diabetes at bay, too.

A look at the eating habits and blood tests of 666 people over age 40 revealed that those who ate salmon every day had a 50 percent lower chance of having glucose intolerance (which includes diabetes and prediabetes) than people who ate that fish less often. In fact, a daily dose of fatty fish may pack as much of a punch as regular exercise or losing weight in staving off diabetes, says Amanda Adler, M.D., Ph.D., study leader and researcher at Seattle Veterans Administration Hospital. But no one should rely solely on fish to ward off the disease, she says.

Researchers got interested in a link between fish and diabetes prevention when they noticed that fish-eating Eskimos got diabetes at much lower rates than their genetic cousins, the Pima Indians. The Pimas have some of the world's highest diabetes rates and rarely eat fish. Researchers think that the fatty acids in the salmon may somehow grease the wheels of the "vans" that deliver glucose into cells. This may prevent what happens in diabetes: Either the vans don't work or the cells can't take the delivery.

It's not clear how the results translate to the rest of the population. But Dr. Adler says that a fish-rich diet probably won't hurt you and may even lower your risk of other diseases. And if salmon and sardines aren't to your taste, mackerel and halibut are rich in fish oils, too.

Once-a-Week Fish Dish Sinks Stroke Risk

Eating fish once or twice a week is looking smarter all the time. Several studies have linked just one serving a week to lower risks of heart disease.

Now a recent study shows that averaging only two-thirds of an ounce of fish a day—any fish—may cut your risk of stroke in half. Since a recommended serving is three ounces, getting one large or two average servings a week should bring you up to a stroke-sparing level.

Red Meat Raises Breast Cancer Threat

Fish or fowl. Either one may help women beat breast cancer. Because when you're eating them, you're not eating the red meat that may multiply your risk of breast cancer by almost two, according to a recent study.

More than 14,000 women were asked about their eating habits, and researchers kept a six-year watch on the women to see who developed breast cancer. Those who said they ate red meat frequently (about once a day) had nearly double the risk of women who said they ate red meat maybe only once a week.

This time, researchers aren't implicating the fat in meat as the main culprit. The fat/breast cancer connection is still a weak one, they say (although there are plenty of other compelling reasons to defat your diet, and even a weak association to breast cancer may be important).

Researchers don't know why red meat may be linked to higher risk. But it's possible that women who eat red meat also tend to do other, yet-to-be-unearthed things that influence their risk for breast cancer. "It may not be fat alone or meat alone or protein alone," says study co-author Paolo Toniolo, M.D., professor of environmental medicine at New York University School of Medicine in New York City. "It may be the complex of dietary habits over a lifetime that influences a woman's hormonal systems."

But that doesn't mean good-eating recommendations change. The point is still to eat meat wisely: Use it as part of a vegetable or carbohydrate dish. Or swap the red stuff for other savory protein options, like easy-to-use soy foods such as tofu and tempeh.

....

Low-Salt Diet a Heart Saver

HAVING A BIG HEART is good for you only if you're dealing in metaphors. In real life, an enlarged heart greatly inflates your risk for heart attacks. But recent research suggests that a good diet might help you get it down to a healthier size—and that it might do the job as well as drugs do.

For a year 76 men and women with enlargement in the heart's left ventricle (usually a consequence of high blood pressure) either cut their sodium intake to 1,600 milligrams a day or stuck to their usual eating habits. (The average American consumes 2,400 to 7,200 milligrams of sodium per day—the equivalent of one to three teaspoons of table salt.) Those who slashed their sodium intake had average reductions in heart enlargement of 5.4 percent.

That's as much as some high blood pressure drugs can do, and it could correspond to a 5 to 10 percent reduction in heart attack risk. Those who didn't change their diets saw no benefits to their heart attack risk profiles.

Salt reduction seems to do something other than just zap high blood pressure. "This study confirms other evidence that the heart is more sensitive to salt intake than blood pressure is," says Richard Devereux, M.D., blood pressure expert and professor of medicine at Cornell University Medical College in New York City. Getting rid of extra salt may reduce the volume of blood that the heart has to pump. And by reducing the workload on the heart, the amount of muscle will go down. "Reversing high salt intake should be a front-line strategy for people with high blood pressure," says Dr. Devereux.

Salt cutbacks here weren't the sort that leave your dinner tasting like cardboard. If you're used to eating an average amount of sodium a day, you might only have to cut out about a teaspoon's worth of salt or less to get the levels used in the study. The easiest place to do that is processed foods—that's where 75 percent of the average diet's sodium is. Only 15 percent comes from what you add at the table. The remaining 10% occurs naturally in nonprocessed foods.

Fortunately, recent changes in labeling laws have made it easier to discern exactly how much sodium certain products contain. A "sodium-free" product must have less than 5 milligrams of sodium per serving, and none of the ingredients can be salt. "Very low sodium" products can't have more than 35 milligrams, but "low sodium" means 140 milligrams or less. "Reduced" and "lite" are less specific—reductions in sodium must be at least 25 and 50 percent, respectively. But beware: Even "reduced-sodium" products can be loaded with the white stuff.

B$_{12}$ Builds Healthier Babies

WE KNOW THAT PREGNANT WOMEN getting plenty of folate, a B vitamin, deliver fewer babies with brain and spinal cord defects. Now a study in Ireland has found that mothers who gave birth to babies with these defects had lower blood levels of another B vitamin, B$_{12}$, than mothers of healthy babies had.

More research is needed to confirm and explain this preliminary finding. But in the meantime, B$_{12}$ expert Joel Mason, M.D., of the Jean Mayer USDA Human Nutrition Research Center on Aging at Tufts University in Boston says that women of childbearing age who eat meat, fish, eggs or dairy foods—the only natural dietary sources of vitamin B$_{12}$—should be getting enough of this vitamin. Strict vegetarians risk a B$_{12}$ deficiency and should consider a supplement, he advises.

Part II

Foods for Better Health

Aging

Eat and Grow Young

THE BUILDING LOOKED almost brand new until someone came along with a wrecking ball.

At first, when the ball started swinging, you didn't see much damage. A window smashed here. A cornice there. A small hole in the roof. Still, how much of this battering could the building take?

Then something peculiar started to happen. After a couple of days of steady pounding, the wrecking ball was doing less damage. It kept swinging away, but now it bounced more often than it landed.

The building, it now appeared, would be safe and sound for a long, long time.

Cell Destroyers—And Defenders

Until recently, researchers didn't understand much about the cellular wrecking balls that threaten good health and youthful living—the antagonistic, submicroscopic cell-wall smashers called free radicals.

Free radicals are really just highly reactive molecules roaming in search of a partner. What makes them so interactive is a purely chemical reaction. That reaction—known as the oxidation process—sets free radicals loose inside our innocent cells.

On the other side, protecting our bodies from the onslaught of these gate crashers, are chemicals and nutrients identified as antioxidants. Some antioxidants occur naturally in our cells; others can be found in some foods.

So how do scientists know that dietary antioxidants are really free radical busters?

By looking at what's *not* visible, says Pamela Starke-Reed, Ph.D., director of the Office of Nutrition at the National Institute on Aging (NIA) in Baltimore. "In the presence of antioxidants, what you do see is much less free radical damage occurring."

The process of cell decay is like margarine going rancid, according to Mohsen Meydani, Ph.D., associate professor of nutrition at Tufts University in Boston and a researcher at the Jean Mayer USDA Human Nutrition Research Center on Aging at the university. Like the fat in margarine, the fats within our cells start to decay—or oxidize—when oxygen reaches them.

"That's how skin wrinkles, the body weakens and muscles lose their youthful tone," Dr. Meydani says. As these changes occur at the cellular level, the immune cells in our bodies also can lose their ability to function. "That's also why older people are more susceptible to infection," he adds.

Your body has defenses, however—built-in enzyme forces that normally keep free radicals at controllable levels. Enzymes are protein molecules that speed up chemical reactions in cells. Without their protection, our bodies would literally spoil at top speed, making us old before our time.

Three of these enzymes work as antioxidants. Through a complex chemical process, the enzymes channel the energies of excess free radicals into harmless substances such as water and ordinary oxygen.

Our bodies usually respond to the presence of increased free radicals by boosting production of the antioxidant enzymes. But our cells need all the help they can get to face free radical assaults. Especially damaging are everyday toxins and pollutants, such as first- and secondhand cigarette smoke, car exhaust fumes and other infamous health wreckers.

Want to Stay Youthful? Get Crunchin'

While you can't spend your life dodging pollutants, you *can* rebuild your natural antioxidant defenses by being selective about the food you eat.

Since antioxidant nutrients are not made in the body like the enzymes, they need to be replenished every day. And that's where a high-antioxidant diet comes in.

Researchers are convinced that three of the most potent and valuable antioxidants are vitamin C, vitamin E and beta-carotene. In a review conducted by the Gerontology Research Center of the NIA, researchers concluded that antioxidant levels in our bodies may help determine how many age-related diseases we have as well as the general status of our health.

Many fruits and vegetables are loaded with antioxidants. But in order to get adequate amounts of antioxidant protection from your diet, you need to eat no fewer than five servings of fruits and vegetables every day, say researchers. Unfortunately, fewer than 10 percent of Americans get this important daily dose of defense.

What happens if you eat lots of flavorful fruits and tender-crisp vegetables? Not only do these foods give you plenty of rejuvenating antioxidants but they also are natural sources of fiber, which helps keep cholesterol at bay and your digestive system in tune. Round out your meals with protein, calcium and zinc—from whole grains, low-fat dairy products and small quantities of lean meat—and you're on your way to a longer, healthier life.

Here's a closer look at the true youth foods.

Load Up on Betas

Beta-carotene, one of the star achievers in the crowd of compounds known as carotenoids, has more than 500 related compounds. Their chemical structure gives them an orange-yellow pigment. But dark green vegetables are also great sources of these compounds (as well as other antioxidants).

Beta-carotene is one of four related compounds called carotenes that are converted to vitamin A in the body. It is the most common carotene in the human food supply, says Robert Russell, M.D., a researcher at the Jean Mayer USDA Human Nutrition Research Center on Aging at Tufts, and it's a vital dietary antioxidant.

Beta-carotene, also known as provitamin A, breaks down into highly active forms of vitamin A, which play an important role in vision, hearing, taste and smell. Best of all, studies have shown that when this hard-working carotene turns into one active vitamin A compound, it fights the free radical damage that causes cancer and heart disease.

Here's how to maximize beta-carotene—and its cousin carotenes—in your diet.

OPT FOR ORANGE. Orange-yellow produce will give you the most generous amounts of beta-carotene, according to

The Beta-Carotene Bull's-Eye

Beta-carotene is an important youth-preserving antioxidant, and just a single daily serving of fruits or vegetables rich in this nutrient may also reduce your risk of heart attack and stroke. In the target below, the best sources are nearest to the bull's-eye.

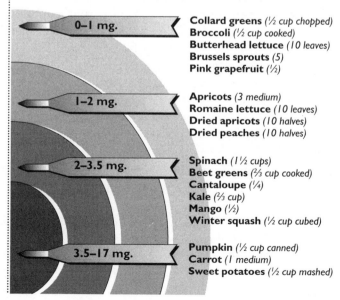

0–1 mg.
Collard greens (½ cup chopped)
Broccoli (½ cup cooked)
Butterhead lettuce (10 leaves)
Brussels sprouts (5)
Pink grapefruit (½)

1–2 mg.
Apricots (3 medium)
Romaine lettuce (10 leaves)
Dried apricots (10 halves)
Dried peaches (10 halves)

2–3.5 mg.
Spinach (1½ cups)
Beet greens (⅔ cup cooked)
Cantaloupe (¼)
Kale (⅔ cup)
Mango (½)
Winter squash (½ cup cubed)

3.5–17 mg.
Pumpkin (½ cup canned)
Carrot (1 medium)
Sweet potatoes (½ cup mashed)

Dr. Russell. While carrots are a great source of beta-carotene, "Don't forget dried apricots, sweet potatoes, red peppers and orange winter squash," he notes. Watermelon and cantaloupe are also good sources, as are broccoli, spinach, kale, turnip greens, beet greens and collard greens.

SEAL IN NUTRIENTS. If you're going to cook carrots, steam them until they're just slightly tender. This increases the availability of their carotene content three- or fourfold without decreasing the benefit of the fiber, according to Dr. Russell. And the availability of beta-carotene in broccoli doubles as soon as that vegetable is lightly cooked. (But don't use enough water to cover the vegetables. You'll end up boiling them and pouring a considerable amount of their carotenes down the drain with the broth.)

EAT MORE PUMPKIN. "Pumpkin has an incredible amount of beta-carotene," Dr. Russell notes. A slice of pumpkin pie or pumpkin bread offers a hefty amount of beta-carotene, so enjoy it for a special dessert. You might also prepare fresh pumpkin and store it, suggests Sooja Kim, R.D., Ph.D., scientific review administrator of the Nutrition Study Section at the National Institutes of Health in Bethesda, Maryland. Cut the pumpkin into chunks, put it into a food processor and grind it, Dr. Kim advises. "It becomes a wonderful puree that you can use fresh or frozen for pumpkin pies or soups." (Canned pumpkin contains virtually the same amount of beta-carotene as fresh pumpkin.)

SUPERCHARGE YOUR SALADS. Iceberg lettuce is a real loser when it comes to carotene counting, according to Dr. Russell. So choose dark, leafy greens such as spinach or Romaine lettuce, which have several times the beta-carotene content of iceberg lettuce. And anytime you add some raw broccoli or a few kale leaves, you're giving your salad a mighty beta boost.

If you have trouble getting used to the more vivid taste of these greens, blend them in with iceberg a bit at a time.

POUR ON THE PUMPKIN. Once you have pumpkin puree in your freezer, you can whip up a quick, scrumptious pumpkin salad dressing in just a minute. "Mix pumpkin puree, oil, vinegar, garlic and your favorite herbs to taste," Dr. Kim recommends. Pour some on your favorite salad—and keep the rest in the fridge for next time.

Also, use pumpkin puree in meat loaf instead of tomato sauce, says Dr. Kim. It's a new, unexpected taste—and utterly delicious.

TRY TROPICAL TEMPTATIONS. Tempt your taste buds with papaya and mango, both rich sources of beta-carotene. Papaya is a deep orange–colored tropical fruit with a very mild flavor that's a cross between honeydew melon and cantaloupe. Just slice it open, remove the seeds and sprinkle it with lime juice to complement its flavor.

Sweeter than papayas, mangoes are delicious sliced on hot cereal. "They're also a popular Thai dessert," Dr. Kim notes. "Just cut up a mango, then mix it with cooked rice, a little brown sugar and lime juice."

For an incredible treat anytime, Dr. Kim recommends a mango "smoothie." Put sliced mango in a blender with a cup of skim milk and a ripe banana and blend until smooth.

Vitamin C: Age Eraser?

Vitamin C is a vital ingredient in the formation of collagen, the biological "glue" that binds your cells together. Vitamin C also helps your body absorb other vital nutrients, such as iron and calcium.

And now there's compelling evidence that vitamin C may be a wellspring of the fountain of youth. Vitamin C is actually your body's first line of defense against early aging. When oxidants are added to human blood, vitamin C is the first antioxidant to cancel them out, before any of the other antioxidants go to work.

In a study at the University of California at Berkeley, researchers removed vitamin C from the blood plasma of healthy volunteers and then added the kinds of oxidants that cause cell breakdown. After the vitamin C was removed, they found oxidation picked up rapidly. But when they put the vitamin C back in, the plasma was again protected from oxidation.

Because vitamin C is water-soluble, it's generally not stored in the body for long. Excess vitamin C is regularly passed in the urine rather than stored away, according to Dr. Starke-Reed.

"Vitamin C is something you have to consume every day by eating citrus fruits and other high-C foods. And the older you get, the more important this behavior is," says Dr. Starke-Reed.

From recent studies it looks as if as little as 300 milligrams a day seems to tilt the scales in our favor. To get that much, you'd need to drink a cup of orange juice and eat one cup of cantaloupe chunks and a one-cup serving of steamed broccoli sometime during the day.

Here are some other ways to keep your cells chock-full of vitamin C.

STOCK YOUR OJ BY THE WEEK. After one week, orange juice that's been opened and stored in its own carton or a plastic pitcher in the fridge loses just 12 percent of its vitamin C,

Keep Vibrant with Vitamin C

Strawberries, grapefruit and broccoli not only delight your palate, they may also "C" you into a longer life. Why? These fruits and vegetables are especially rich in super-antioxidant vitamin C. And a large study from the University of California School of Public Health in Los Angeles has shown that consuming more vitamin C may reward you with more years of life.

A total of 11,348 adults participated in the national nutrition survey. Three groups of men and women were tracked for an average of 15 years. Group one took in less than 50 milligrams of vitamin C each day from food, group two took in about 150 milligrams daily (also from food) and group three

say researchers from the U.S. Citrus and Subtropical Products Laboratory in Winter Haven, Florida. But after two weeks, the loss jumps to around 35 percent. If you drink one small cup of orange juice daily, buy just a quart. Better yet, squeeze your own when you need it! And if you mix your juice from frozen concentrate, fix small batches regularly for maximum C. When used promptly, other fresh or frozen juices contain similar levels of vitamin C (about 120 milligrams per cup), so just enjoy your favorite.

VARY YOUR SALAD ROUTINE. Add orange and grapefruit sections to your green salads. Or opt for all-fruit salads, using plenty of cantaloupe and honeydew melon, strawberries and kiwifruit in addition to citrus.

PICK PEPPERS. Both red and green peppers are a good source of vitamin C, but the reds pack more than double the antioxidant of the green variety. Include sliced peppers in your snack pack for home, car or office or enjoy them with your favorite low-fat dip.

---

got a total of over 300 milligrams from both food and supplement sources.

Over the 15-year span of the study, researchers found that the high-C men in group three had a much lower death rate than the low-C men from group one. In fact, judging from this study, men who get plenty of vitamin C in their diets can expect to live 6 years longer than those who consume very little.

Women also benefit from C, though less dramatically, according to the study. The women in group three—the ones who got over 300 milligrams a day from food and supplements—averaged a two-year longer life span than those in group one.

Hitting Free Radicals Where They Live

Vitamin E may be the most powerful nutrient there is for preventing chronic illness and premature aging, researchers say. Vitamin E is so promising that numerous studies are under way to determine exactly what it does and how it works. Already the news is good.

Vitamin E behaves like the Wild West sheriff of your cells, shooting it out with free radicals before they stake their claim to your cells. When you are exposed to a variety of environmental carcinogens, ranging from tobacco smoke and pesticides to ozone and radiation, the oxidation process picks up its pace and increases your risk of cancer. But several studies now suggest that vitamin E meets these toxic compounds at the boundaries of your cells and may prevent them from causing cancerous tumors.

Take ozone, for example, which is a key component of smog. In a laboratory experiment, researchers at the New England Medical Center in Boston exposed cells pretreated with vitamin E to ozone and demonstrated that vitamin E made the cells resistant to free radical attack.

That's how vitamin E seems to protect cells most, other studies indicate. It helps keep cell walls intact so that toxins can't enter, and it makes it hard for free radicals to swoop in.

Vitamin E also boosts your immune power—and that's a vital part of your body's defenses against cancer. One study directed by Dr. Meydani at the Human Nutrition Research Center at Tufts showed that vitamin E supplements clearly improved the immune response in healthy adults. This finding is believed to be particularly important, because our immune system usually weakens as we age.

Because vitamin E has an antioxidant action, researchers also think that it could help ease youth-sapping rheumatoid arthritis—and some animal studies seem to confirm this. When people have this kind of arthritis, it's because free radical molecules have rushed to the aching joint, attracted by the presence of bacteria. And those free radicals produce painful inflammation. But if you get plenty of vitamin E, researchers surmise, you may be able to reduce the effects of arthritis as you age.

Researchers are also trying to find out whether vitamin E (and other powerful antioxidants) can help prevent or alleviate certain kinds of cancers and some common problems of aging, such as Parkinson's disease and cataracts.

Easy Ways to Get Your E

Food sources might give you all the vitamin E you need to maintain health, but they're not a sure thing. The Daily Value (DV) is 30 international units per day—and some diets do provide that much.

There's a problem with food sources, however. Vitamin E tends to hang out in some unsavory places—chiefly in foods that contain polyunsaturated fat. Nuts, dairy products, eggs and certain vegetable oils are prime examples of high-fat foods that contain an abundance of vitamin E. And eating too many fatty foods promotes obesity, warns Dr. Meydani.

To get the full benefits of this powerhouse nutrient, you may want to ask your doctor about supplements, suggests Dr. Meydani. For most people, a daily dose of 100 to 400 international units would help promote health and longevity.

But even if you do take supplements, there are other ways to get vitamin E in your diet without overdoing your daily fat intake. Here are some tactics that get the nod from nutritionists.

SEED YOUR SALADS. Sprinkle a few sunflower seeds over your salads, suggests Dr. Kim. They're rich in vitamin E.

TOAST A HEALTHY TREAT. If you're eating more antioxidant-rich pumpkin, don't toss the seeds! They're chock-full of vitamin E and easy to prepare for snacks. Just wash and dry the seeds, then scatter them onto a baking sheet and roast at 150° until they're crunchy.

Peanuts and almonds are good sources of vitamin E, too, but as with sunflower seeds, you should go easy because of the fat content. "As always, moderation is the best policy," cautions Dr. Kim.

(continued on page 33)

The Longevity Menu

How easy is it to pack age-erasing antioxidants into your daily life? Very.

To get started, try this three-day, high-antioxidant plan. Every meal includes foods that are good sources

DAY 1

BREAKFAST

1 cup crisped rice cereal with 1 cup skim milk
1 mixed-grain English muffin with 1 teaspoon
    margarine
1 pear

LUNCH

Sandwich made with 2 slices mixed-grain bread,
    3 ounces smoked turkey breast, 2 leaves iceberg
    lettuce, 2 tablespoons low-fat mayonnaise and
    ½ sliced tomato
2 kiwifruits
6 ounces low-fat fruit yogurt

DINNER

3 ounces broiled beef tenderloin
1 cup cooked long-grain brown rice
Salad made with ½ cup Romaine lettuce,
    ½ tomato, 1 slice avocado and 2 tablespoons
    Italian dressing
1 cup cooked broccoli
2 slices enriched whole-wheat bread with
    2 teaspoons margarine
1 cup skim milk

Antioxidant analysis: 333.9 mg. vitamin C, 32.8 IU vitamin E, 1.5 mg. beta-carotene

of vitamin C, vitamin E and beta-carotene. For the vegetables and fruits in any of these meals, you can substitute other antioxidant-rich varieties, such as strawberries, cantaloupe, kale and spinach.

DAY 2

BREAKFAST

1 cup bran nuggets cereal with 3 tablespoons raisins and 1 cup skim milk
2 slices enriched wheat toast with 2 teaspoons margarine
½ papaya
1 cup skim milk

LUNCH

1 cup 1% low-fat cottage cheese
½ pear
½ peach
2 whole-wheat rolls with 2 teaspoons margarine and 2 tablespoons jam or preserves

DINNER

3 ounces broiled haddock
1 cup mashed sweet potatoes
Salad made with loose leaf lettuce, ¼ cup chopped raw mushrooms, ¼ cup diced tomato and 2 tablespoons blue cheese dressing
1 cup skim milk

Antioxidant analysis: 244 mg. vitamin C, 29.9 IU vitamin E, 23.5 mg. beta-carotene

(continued)

The Longevity Menu—Continued

DAY 3

BREAKFAST

½ cup all-bran cereal with ½ cup sliced banana
and I cup skim milk
½ cup fresh-squeezed orange juice
I cinnamon roll with icing

LUNCH

Sandwich made with I whole-wheat roll, 2 ounces
smoked deli ham, I ounce low-fat Swiss cheese
and 2 tablespoons low-fat mayonnaise
½ cup canned plums in light syrup
½ mango
½ cup canned sweetened grapefruit juice

DINNER

3 ounces baked salmon
2 whole-wheat rolls with 2 tablespoons
margarine
½ cup baby lima beans
Salad with ¼ head iceberg lettuce, ¼ cup raw
carrots, ¼ cup chopped spinach and
2 tablespoons Russian dressing
I cup skim milk
½ cup cooked dried apricots

Antioxidant analysis: 207.3 mg. vitamin C, 35.8 IU
vitamin E, 9.2 mg. beta-carotene.

EAT WHEAT GERM. This vitamin- and mineral-rich embryo of the wheat berry contains four milligrams of vitamin E per quarter-cup. Try it toasted or raw on frozen yogurt. Wheat germ also makes a healthy addition to casseroles, meat loaf, bread, muffins and pancakes.

Two More Youth Extenders

A youthful body deserves a sturdy frame—and that means getting plenty of calcium in your diet. But along with calcium, you need plenty of vitamin D. Without it your bones won't harden no matter how much calcium you offer them. And although neither calcium nor vitamin D is an antioxidant, they are still top "youth nutrients."

You can get plenty of vitamin D in your diet from a variety of low-fat products. Nonfat milk, along with many breads and cereals, is usually fortified with D. Just two cups of fortified skim milk supplies 50 percent of the DV for vitamin D.

Experts recommend that most people get at least 1,000 milligrams of calcium a day. Exceptions: Men and women under age 25 should get 1,200 milligrams per day, and the National Osteoporosis Foundation recommends that postmenopausal women aim for 1,500 milligrams daily if they're not on estrogen replacement therapy.

The best sources of calcium by far are nonfat or low-fat dairy products. Several are fortified with vitamin D, which makes it easy to get both vital bone builders at once. Eight ounces of nonfat yogurt, for instance, offer 452 milligrams of calcium, while a cup of skim milk has 302 milligrams.

Sardines also offer rich amounts of calcium because you eat the tiny calcium-rich bones in the sardines. Just seven sardines provide 321 milligrams of calcium. Similarly, three ounces of pink salmon, with bones, supply 181 milligrams.

Once you turn to plant sources, the calcium numbers start to slide, but vegetables still offer good amounts of this mineral. Half-cup servings of Chinese cabbage (bok choy), mustard greens, kale and pinto beans have amounts ranging from 41 to 86 milligrams.

Allergy Relief
What's Eating You?
Could Be What You're Eating

THINK YOU HAVE A FOOD ALLERGY? If so, you're among the more than one-fourth of adult Americans convinced that some of the foods they bite into wind up biting them back. But despite the widespread worry, "True food allergies are quite rare, probably affecting less than 1 percent of the adult population," says Hugh Sampson, M.D., professor of pediatrics, allergy and immunology at Johns Hopkins University Medical Center in Baltimore.

Does this mean that you don't have a food allergy? Not necessarily. "But it's more likely that a person who thinks he or she has a food allergy actually has a food intolerance," says allergist-immunologist Wesley A. Burks, M.D., associate professor of pediatrics at the University of Arkansas for Medical Sciences in Little Rock. Food intolerances—lactose intolerance is the most well-known example—can be quite nasty in their own right. "Food intolerances produce some of the same uncomfortable symptoms that food allergies create, including bloating, cramping, gas and diarrhea," says Dr. Burks.

Anatomy of an Allergy

An allergy is the body's abnormal reaction to a harmless substance. Even the healthiest foods may trigger a reaction in susceptible persons. Ironically, it's your body's immune system—designed to protect you from naughty invaders—that accounts for the symptoms. Histamine and other chemicals released from specialized calls called mast cells cause a wide range of allergic symptoms. Food allergy symptoms can appear for the first time in adulthood. "Why allergies strike when they do remains a mystery," says Dr. Burks.

An intolerance can be from a direct effect of some food or a deficiency of some enzyme, as in the case of lactose intolerance, where the enzyme lactase is deficient. And, like allergies, intolerances can also strike for the first time in adulthood.

Knowing the difference between allergies and intolerances can be critical: Intolerances are often controlled by limiting the amount of the food eaten; with allergies, total avoidance is the rule. "Allergies are potentially fatal when they cause an anaphylactic reaction," says Dean Metcalfe, M.D., head of the allergic diseases section of the Laboratory of Clinical Investigation at the National Institute of Allergy and Infectious Diseases (a division of the National Institutes of Health) in Bethesda, Maryland. Anaphylactic reactions are characterized by severe itching, hives, sweating, swelling of the throat, difficulty breathing and a sudden, severe drop in blood pressure sometimes leading to loss of consciousness. If not treated immediately with epinephrine (adrenaline), anaphylactic shock can result in death. People with asthma appear to be at special risk. Anyone who has ever experienced an allergic reaction to a food should carry a kit to self-administer epinephrine. These kits must be prescribed by a physician.

Figuring out whether you actually have a food allergy or intolerance or tracking down the culprit food isn't easy. Just consider the sheer number of foods and ingredients that you ingest at every meal. Even a simple breakfast can leave you asking "Was it the cereal? The milk? Or the banana slices on top?"

But rest assured, you can find answers—and relief. The following quiz leads you step-by-step through the key questions that leading allergists ask to discover whether you really do have a food allergy, a food intolerance or neither. It's intended for adults, not children, and is not meant as a substitute for seeing your doctor. Its main purpose is to help you get the information that you and your doctor need to arrive at a conclusive diagnosis. If you have any type of severe reaction following a meal, however—such as difficulty breathing—you should contact your doctor immediately.

So simply answer the questions and tally your scores at the end of each section. Depending on the numbers, you may be asked to skip ahead to another section. As you work your way through, you might discover some very useful clues. The next step is a firm diagnosis—and only your doctor can provide that.

Part I: Allergy, Intolerance or Toxin?

1. **Do you have asthma?**
    YES ___ 1   NO ___ 0

    If you have asthma, you are not only at greater risk for food allergies but also for anaphylactic reactions, which can be life-threatening. (See "Have Allergies? Avoid These Food Additives" on page 41.)

2. **Did anyone eating with you get sick or experience unusual feelings at the same time?**
    YES ___ 0   NO ___ 1

    If others who ate the same meal also felt sick, it's very likely that you ate a contaminated food. Chief culprits are undercooked or improperly stored fish, meat, poultry, dairy and egg products.

3. **Did your discomfort begin within 45 minutes of eating?**
    YES ___ 1   NO ___ 0

    "Most allergic reactions occur within 45 minutes after ingesting the food," says Dr. Metcalfe, "and some reactions may be immediate." So if your reaction is delayed by hours, you're probably dealing with a food intolerance, not an allergy.

    After the initial allergic response, which may occur within seconds or minutes, other symptoms may occur over several hours.

4. Do you have nonfood allergies?

YES ___ 1   NO ___ 0

"Most food allergies develop in allergic individuals," says Dr. Metcalfe. "If you're allergic to begin with—if you have been allergic to cats or ragweed, for example—you are at higher risk for developing a food allergy." Asthma and chronic skin conditions such as eczema can be exacerbated by food allergies.

Total points _____

Assessment
  0 to 1 point: Food allergy unlikely; possibility of food intolerance. *Skip to "Part 4: Food Intolerance," on page 42.*
  2 to 3 points: Possibility of food allergy.
  4 points: Good chance of food allergy.

This is a preliminary screening to narrow the possibilities. Next you'll look at specific symptoms.

Part 2: Allergic Symptoms

5. Does your mouth itch after eating a suspect food?

YES ___ 5   NO ___ 0

This is often the first symptom of an allergic reaction because the lips, tongue, palate and throat are the first to come in contact with a food. When these areas react, this group of symptoms is sometimes called oral allergy syndrome.

This syndrome is far more common in allergic people and has been likened to specific foods including watermelon, cantaloupe, honeydew and bananas. So if you experience oral allergy syndrome in reaction to these or any other foods, it's likely you're allergic.

6. **Does your nose run and do your eyes water after eating a nonspicy food?**

   YES ___ 1   NO ___ 0

   These symptoms of allergic rhinitis can occur with food allergies. But the symptoms can also result from eating spicy foods, in which case it is called gustatory rhinitis, which has nothing to do with an allergic reaction.

7. **Do you break out in a rash after eating certain foods?**

   YES ___ 1   NO ___ 0

   Hives or skin rashes are among the most common allergic reactions to foods. However, skin reactions have a wide variety of cases beyond food allergies. And while food allergies frequently cause acute hives, they are rarely responsible for chronic hives.

8. **Do you experience frequent crying spells?**

   YES ___ 0   NO ___ 0

   While nutrition may be related to emotional health, emotional reactions have not been scientifically linked to food allergy.

9. **Do you have irritable bowel syndrome?**

   YES ___ 0   NO ___ 0

   Though careful attention to diet may be crucial to overcoming this condition, irritable bowel syndrome has not been scientifically linked to food allergy.

10. **Do you have difficulty breathing after eating certain foods?**

    YES ___ 2   NO ___ 0

    A food allergen can affect breathing both through swelling of the windpipe and through its effects on the lungs. People with asthma are at special risk. However, there can be multiple triggers for an asthmatic attack besides foods.

11. Do you suffer from migraine headaches?

YES ___ 0   NO ___ 0

Migraines are not likely to be caused by food allergies, A substance called tyramine, however, found in red wine and aged cheeses, may trigger migraines in susceptible people. But this is a direct chemical reaction, not an immune system allergy.

12. Do you suffer from chronic fatigue?

YES ___ 0   NO ___ 0

Though an individual's diet plays a role in overall energy levels, chronic fatigue has not been scientifically linked to food allergy.

13. Do you have abdominal pain after eating certain foods?

YES ___ 1   NO ___ 0

Bloating, cramping, gas and diarrhea are symptoms shared by allergies and food intolerance.

Total points _____

Assessment: While several of the above symptoms could be a sign of food allergy, no single symptom tells us very much. "What we're looking for," says Dr. Burks, "are symptom *clusters.*"

For example, abdominal pain can be a symptom of allergy or intolerance. But when that pain is accompanied by a runny nose or skin rash, allergy becomes a far greater probability.

0 to 1 point: Food allergy unlikely. *Skip to "Part 4: Food Intolerance," on page 42.*

2 to 4 points: Possibility of food allergy.

5 to 10 points: Strong chance of food allergy.

Part 3: Food Allergy Suspects

The following foods can cause allergy in some people.

Walnuts. Walnuts and other tree nuts—Brazil nuts, almonds, cashews, pistachios, filberts (hazelnuts), pecans, hickory nuts, pine nuts—are among the most allergenic foods. If you are allergic to one tree nut variety, there is a chance you're allergic to others—but not necessarily to peanuts, which are legumes.

Peanuts. Though peanuts can be a healthy addition to most diets, they are also among the most allergenic of all foods. In severely allergic persons, just a fraction of a peanut kernel can be enough to set off a reaction.

Shrimp and other shellfish. Although shrimp gets much attention, a broad class of shellfish can cause an allergic reaction. This class includes other crustacea (lobster, crab and prawn) and mollusks (snails, mussels, oysters, scallops, clams, squid and octopus).

Finfish. Compared with other major food allergens, the proteins in fish are more vulnerable to heat and other forms of preparation. So some persons allergic to fresh cooked salmon or tuna can eat canned salmon or tuna without difficulty. But don't count on it.

In extremely severe fish allergies, even inhaling the vapors from boiling fish can set off a reaction.

Reactions to toxins in fish are sometimes mistaken for fish allergies. Scromboid poisoning from fish occurs when fish are contaminated with high levels of histamine, the primary irritant in classic allergic reactions.

Milk and milk products. Most adverse reactions to milk are not allergies but rather lactose intolerance. Knowing the difference is critical: Those with lactose intolerance can generally manage small amounts of milk; with true milk allergy, *any* consumption of milk or milk-related proteins can be dangerous.

Tofu and soy foods. Tofu is made from soy, a major allergen in children. Some adults react, too.

Wheat-containing foods. Wheat allergy should not be

confused with celiac disease (often called celiac sprue), a rare condition resulting from an intolerance to gluten, which is present not only in wheat, but also in rye, barley and oats.

Assessment: The foods in Part 3 top the list of suspects. The first four mentioned "account for 90 percent of all food allergies," says Dr. Sampson. So if you think that you've consistently reacted to one of these foods, (multiple allergies are rare), the odds are good that you have a true food allergy.

Skip to "Part 5: Your Diet Diary," on page 44.

Have Asthma? Avoid These Food Additives

Reactions to food additives are even more rare than food allergies. However, for two groups of people —those with asthma and those with chronic skin conditions—certain food additives can bring a significant, if small, chance of reaction.

Sulfites. Sulfites are compounds used in foods as preservatives. Four percent of people with asthma react to sulfites. These persons are at risk for anaphylactic reactions. The problem comes from the release of sulfur dioxide gas, which may trigger a fall in pulmonary (lung) function. Sulfites appear under the names *sodium sulfite, sodium-* or *potassium bisulfite* or *metabisulfites.*

Monosodium glutamate (MSG). People with asthma appear more at risk for reactions to MSG.

Food coloring. In people with chronic hives, reaction to certain food colorings is probably on the order of 5 to 10 percent. The greatest offenders appear to be the so-called azo dyes, which include FD&C red #4 (ponceau), FD&C yellow #6 (monoazo) and FD&C yellow #5 (tartrazine). Tartrazine is also suspected of exacerbating asthma, though the jury is still out.

Part 4: Food Intolerance

The following foods can cause food intolerance.

Carbohydrates. Even if you don't have a food allergy, foods could be causing you trouble—even the healthiest of foods. In fact, a surprising culprit has been identified in the past few years: carbohydrates.

One type of carbohydrate, fiber, has long been known to cause gastrointestinal distress, often in those who have just begun eating a high-fiber diet. That's not surprising, because fiber is not digested on its trip through the small intestine. What is surprising are the recent indications that nonfiber carbohydrates—some sugars and starches—are not completely absorbed before reaching the colon. This is caused by either a simple overload or a deficiency of key enzymes.

The symptoms can be just as unpleasant as food allergy reactions, ranging from uncomfortable abdominal distension, gas and cramps to debilitating chronic diarrhea. Ironically, because many of the foods involved are so healthful, no one would ever suspect them as the source of trouble. If you do seem to react to them, you can first try incorporating them gradually into your diet over a course of weeks. But if you still have problems, limit your intake.

Milk. Milk and milk products contain a sugar, lactose, that is difficult for many people to digest. Lactose intolerance is caused by a lack of lactase, the enzyme that breaks down lactose. When unabsorbed lactose enters the colon, it starts causing trouble: "abdominal bloating, excessive gas production and pain from abdominal distension," says Dr. Metcalfe. These symptoms may be delayed two to eight hours.

Lactose intolerance is prevalent among African-Americans, Native Americans and people of Hispanic, Asian or Mediterranean descent. Many people who've consumed little milk since childhood and begin drinking it again once they hit age 40 to help fight off osteoporosis encounter an unpleasant surprise: Lactase deficiency can develop during adulthood.

Fruit juices. Fruit juices are high in fructose, a type of sugar touted in recent years as a healthy alternative to sucrose (common table sugar). Unfortunately, fructose is not as easily absorbed as other sugars, and this can lead to abdominal distress.

Apple juice also contains another potential troublemaker: sorbitol, a polyalcohol sugar. The fructose-sorbitol combination is a double whammy: Both together may lead to greater gastrointestinal trouble than either alone.

Sugar-free candies. Sorbitol is the primary sweetener used in many sugar-free candies and gum. Even small amounts may lead to malabsorption and gastrointestinal distress.

Sweetened soft drinks. Most nondiet drinks contain high-fructose corn syrup (HFCS), which may add up to as much as 15 grams of fructose in an eight-ounce glass. Among the soft drinks loaded with HFCS are the so-called natural drinks.

Foods That Contain Lactose

Lactose intolerance is the most common of all food intolerances. The following foods all contain the offending sugar lactose.

HIGH LACTOSE
- Milk, including whole, low-fat, skim, condensed, evaporated, dried and buttermilk
- Frozen yogurt
- Ice cream, sherbet, ice milk
- Mozzarella cheese
- Cottage cheese
- Other soft cheeses

SOME LACTOSE
- Cheeses, including American, Swiss, Cheddar, Parmesan and cream cheese
- Butter
- Margarine
- Yogurt

Fresh fruits. Fruit is a major source of free fructose in the diet. And sorbitol is found in apples, pears, peaches and prunes. If you think you're susceptible to this type of food intolerance, don't eat too much at once.

Beans. As mentioned, high-fiber foods are known to cause bloating and gas in some people. And beans are naturally high in fiber. But in addition, some people may actually suffer from a bean intolerance. New research shows that maldigestion of the starch component of beans may also contribute to distress. Add fiber to the diet slowly or limit it if this go-slow approach doesn't help.

Part 5: Your Diet Diary

A diet diary is a record of everything you eat, the time you eat it, the amount and any symptoms that occur throughout the day. By examining the diet diary, you and your doctor may be able to spot unforeseen relationships between symptoms and the foods you have eaten. If you've answered the relevant questions in this worksheet, and you think you may indeed have a food allergy, consider keeping a food diary for one to two weeks. Then take it with you when you see your doctor.

Here are some tips to help you get the most useful information from your food diary.

- Carry it with you at all times; don't wait until the end of the day to fill it in.
- Write down everything that enters your mouth, including beverages, medicines and even chewing gum.
- Indicate when any symptoms began and how long they lasted.
- Be very specific. For example, don't write "ham sandwich," but instead list all the ingredients: "smoked ham, white bread, brown mustard . . . "
- Whenever possible, attach ingredient labels to your food diary as a handy quick reference for your doctor. (Labels are extremely helpful when considering food additives.)

Even with a careful record of everything you eat, the data can sometimes fool you. So once you have identified a food as a potential suspect, you and your doctor will need to consider the following questions:

Did you react to the suspect food every time? This is considered powerful evidence of a food-related problem, allergy or intolerance. It's not conclusive, however, so your doctor will need to confirm your suspicions with a skin-prick test.

If you don't react to the food every time, that doesn't always mean the food is innocent. In fact, there are several reasons that your reaction to a food allergen may appear erratic.

How much of the suspect food did you eat? "The most likely reason you wouldn't react every time is in the amount you're eating," says Dr. Metcalfe. "If you eat a little, you may not react; if you eat a lot, you may react.

"Say you ate lobster once and reacted, and then found that the salad you just ate had lobster in it, but you didn't

What Bananas and Rubber Have in Common

Sometimes a person who is allergic to one food is allergic to other related foods—or even to nonfoods. If you're allergic to a plant listed below, you may also react to the substances listed after it.

• Ragweed—Watermelon, cantaloupe, honeydew, bananas, chamomile tea, sunflower seeds
• Mugwort—Celery
• Birch pollen—Carrots, apples, hazelnuts, potatoes
• Bananas—Latex

If you're allergic to one food in the following families, you may be allergic to another.

• Shellfish—Lobster, crab, prawn, shrimp
• Legumes—Peas, beans, soybeans, peanuts

react. That doesn't mean you're not allergic. The key may be in the amount consumed."

Do you drink alcohol? The ingestion of alcohol increases the absorption of food allergens. So if you take a drink, you're more susceptible to an allergic reaction. That means you may react to some food only after you've consumed it with alcohol.

Did you exercise after you ate? In susceptible people, exercise can cause an allergic reaction to a food eaten before the exercise session. For some, the allergic reaction occurs in response to particular foods. Though rare, exercise-induced food allergy can be quite serious. Some people will have an anaphylactic reaction only after exercising. But prevention is simple; before exercising, just don't eat any food that you suspect of causing a problem.

Part 6: Living with Food Allergy

Discovering that you have a true food allergy is a double-edged sword. On the one hand, it means always needing to be aware of what you're eating. On the other hand, knowing for sure lets you take steps to put an end to troubling symptoms—and maybe even save your life.

In about one-third of adult food allergies, reactions to the allergen disappear within one to two years following complete avoidance. However, the development of tolerance depends on the food, with the major allergens—peanuts in particular—least likely to relinquish their hold.

"In adults it's simply not reliable to stop eating a food and hope your allergy will not come back," says Dr. Metcalfe. "I think once you're allergic to a food, it's safest to assume you're allergic to that food for the rest of your life."

The toughest part of living with a food allergy is that even once you know what to look out for, actually finding it can be difficult. That's because the same food can be disguised under different names. For example, lactalbumin is a milk protein.

If it's tough deciphering label ingredients listed, it's impossible to detect ingredients that aren't. Food and Drug Administration regulations require the listing of only those ingredients that make up 2 percent or more of a food product. Unfortunately, this seemingly small amount may be more than enough to set off an allergic reaction for some sensitive people.

Even when you think you know the ingredients in a product, labels change. "So you must always check, even when you think you know," says Anne Munoz-Furlong, founder and president of the Food Allergy Network in Fairfax, Virginia. Also, be advised that food products imported from other countries may not be subject to the same disclosure standards.

If food labels are daunting, cafeterias and restaurants can be precarious. Since there are no labels to read, you have to count on the reliability of the chef to let you know the full ingredients in any menu selection. Munoz-Furlong has this advice: "Speak with the restaurant manager rather than relying on your waiter or waitress. And don't ever be afraid to ask questions!" One of the best questions: What other foods have been prepared on the same grill? If an allergic food has been cooked earlier, small amounts of cross-contamination could infiltrate your meal.

....

Arthritis
Try This Ache-Away Diet

THE ALARM SOUNDS. Rescue trucks rush to the scene, loaded with special flame-fighting chemicals.

In the first few moments of confusion, it looks like the emergency is well in hand. As the rescue team pours on the fire-dousing chemicals, the fire is reduced to embers.

But what's this? Even while the owner is congratulating the firefighters on a job well-done, things start to go wrong with the building. Doors that once opened easily are now stiff and creaky. Windows that once moved up and down smoothly are now groaning. All those exotic chemicals saved

the building, only to attack the hinges and joints of the vener-
able structure.

Time for repairs.

When a Rescue Goes Awry

Like the chemicals that save the building but damage the
joints and hinges, your body's immune system sometimes
starts a rescue operation that later goes wrong. Cells that fight
inflammation rush to the site of the problem—typically a knee
or an elbow—but in the process of putting out the fire, they
start to whittle away at the cushioning membrane in the joint.
Pretty soon there's a new problem—rheumatoid arthritis—
causing nasty inflammation and pain in susceptible joints.

Rheumatoid isn't the only kind of arthritis. All in all, there
are over 100 types, each dishing out its own brand of misery
and discomfort. Some have known causes, while the origin of
others remains unknown.

Osteoarthritis is much more common than rheumatoid
arthritis, affecting about 60 percent of all arthritis sufferers, or
28 million Americans. Caused by the gradual wearing away of
cartilage—the tough material that protects and cushions the
bones of a joint—osteoarthritis can cause pain in the joints a
number of different ways. For example, pain can result from
damage to the bone or damage to the ligaments that hold the
bones together.

Gout is a form of arthritis most common among middle-
aged men, launching sneak attacks of excruciating pain. The
cause is well-known: People with gout build up uric acid—a
waste product in the blood—and when that crystallizes in a
joint, it causes intense inflammation.

At one time experts believed that there was nothing you
could do for any of these forms of arthritis but take aspirin, rub
on a little ice and learn to live with it. But today rheumatologists (doctors who specialize in treating arthritis and related
diseases) are reevaluating the rules of treatment. And for two
kinds of arthritis—rheumatoid arthritis and gout—doctors
have found that a change in diet can often help bring relief.

Might Diet Ease the Pain?

Although there is no agreement about a diet to fight rheumatoid arthritis, many researchers say that specific changes in diet can help reduce or prevent arthritis pain in certain people.

"Some people may have a favorable response to a specific diet, but that doesn't mean everyone else will," says Jeffrey R. Lisse, M.D., associate professor of medicine and director of the Division of Rheumatology at the University of Texas Medical Branch at the University of Texas Medical School at Galveston. "There are a few studies suggesting that some patients with rheumatic diseases may indeed be diet- or food-sensitive and that this triggers their arthritis flare-ups." But Dr. Lisse emphasizes that there is no single diet that will help large groups of people.

An Easy Way to Go Fish

Many studies have shown that a diet high in omega-3 fatty acids can significantly reduce the inflammation and stiffness associated with rheumatoid arthritis. In most of these studies, participants consumed fish oil containing about three to five grams of omega-3's per day, the equivalent of 8 to 13 ounces of mackerel. Fortunately, there's another way to get your omega-3's: Just take fish oil capsules, which are available over the counter at almost any pharmacy.

That's good news, but doctors are quick to point out that fish oil supplements are not a total substitute for the real McCoy. Fish is a low-fat, nutrient-rich food source that should be a staple of most arthritis patients' diets, says Joel M. Kremer, M.D., professor of medicine and head of the Division of Rheumatology at Albany Medical College in New York. And frequent use of fish oil capsules can cause gas.

A healthful, balanced diet is the only one that is consistently helpful to most people, he says. He recommends that you talk to your doctor before embarking on any diet plan that calls for the elimination of large groups of foods or that relies heavily on only a few foods.

But while special diets don't provide the answer for most people who have rheumatoid arthritis, other doctors agree that overall good nutrition is definitely a factor in keeping this disease under control.

"There is no doubt that what you eat can modify the function of your immune system," says David S. Pisetsky, M.D., Ph.D., medical adviser to the Arthritis Foundation and author of *The Duke University Medical Center Book of Arthritis*.

Conversely, poor eating habits can cause the immune system to go on the fritz. "Foods are clearly linked to a variety of immune-mediated inflammatory reactions such as asthma and hives," says Dr. Pisetsky. "It would not be surprising if rheumatoid arthritis as well as other forms of arthritis in some people resulted from a similar immune response."

Dr. Pisetsky recommends that people with arthritis should eat a variety of foods and try to maintain their ideal weight by eating a low-fat diet. Staying at that weight, Dr. Pisetsky points out, allows the immune system to get all the nutritional benefits it needs. And he says a low-fat weight-loss plan can help stave off bouts of inflammation.

Weigh Less, Ache Less

Maintaining ideal weight is especially important for someone who has osteoarthritis, the kind that results from the wearing down of cartilage. Researchers have noted that most cases of osteoarthritis start becoming evident in middle age or later years—which is the same time that most of us begin packing on the pounds. And osteoarthritis is even more likely for those who have been carrying extra weight for longer periods of time—since childhood or young adulthood. Extra body weight places extra stress on your joints.

Joint cartilage eventually breaks down when the stress of

moving a load that's too heavy is concentrated in a small area such as the joints, says Kenneth D. Brandt, M.D., professor of medicine and head of the rheumatology division at Indiana University School of Medicine in Indianapolis. "Losing just a few pounds can significantly reduce that load and improve the way people feel."

In a long-term Framingham Knee Osteoarthritis study, researchers selected 796 women to study over a ten-year period. The researchers found that those who lost an average of 11 pounds—and kept it off—decreased their risk of developing osteoarthritis by over 50 percent.

In studying groups of obese people (people who are 20 percent over their ideal weight), researchers have shown that weight reduction may reduce pain not only in the knees but also in other joints such as the hips, spine and back. It's possible that the excess weight causes changes in the joint cartilage in the body.

And while weight control has been shown to benefit people who have osteoarthritis, it can also help those who have gout. Studies show that the likelihood of recurring gout attacks decreases as people lose pounds.

The Role of Food Allergies

Doctors once scoffed at the notion that food allergies could cause flare-ups. But studies have confirmed that some people definitely have allergies that connect with arthritis in some way.

In one landmark study, researchers at the University of Florida in Gainesville tested a woman who claimed that her rheumatoid arthritis acted up whenever she had milk. They filled some food capsules with freeze-dried milk powder and others with nondairy food powder. All the capsules looked the same.

When the woman ate the nondairy food capsules, she had no increase in her arthritis symptoms. When she took the milk-powder capsules, on the other hand, symptoms of morning stiffness, joint swelling and joint tenderness increased, peaking 24 to 48 hours later. In the study, researchers repeated the test four times, and the results were confirmed each time.

Subsequent studies have yielded similar results for some people with allergies to milk as well as other foods. Nevertheless, the percentage of people with arthritis who react this way is very small. One expert estimates that only about 5 percent of those with rheumatoid arthritis are food-sensitive.

Joint Inflamers to Avoid

Among the foods that frequently produce reactions in people with rheumatoid arthritis are many that are high in nutrients. So before you drop any food group from your diet, be sure to talk to your doctor to find out whether you'll need supplements to make up for lost nutrients.

If you decide to go on an elimination diet—that is, eliminating nearly all foods and then gradually reintroducing food groups one at a time—read "Put Your Diet to the Test" on page 54 to find out how to do it. Here are some actions you might want to take if you think your problems are associated with some of the foods you commonly eat.

AVOID TOMATOES. In a dietary study conducted in Israel by researchers at the Golda Medical Center, tomatoes caused symptoms in 22 percent of the patients who had rheumatoid arthritis. If you find that you have to avoid tomatoes, you'll also have to stay away from ketchup, tomato sauce and other products that contain tomatoes. Also, be sure to check labels on soups and prepared foods.

STEER CLEAR OF RED MEAT. People who are allergic to red meat may need to avoid all kinds—pork, lamb and game meats as well as beef. This may seem like a loss at first, until you get used to a vegetarian diet. If you do find that red meat is part of the problem, be sure to look at the plan for switching to a vegetarian diet on page 56.

STAY AWAY FROM DAIRY PRODUCTS. In the dietary study in Israel, researchers also found that milk caused symptoms in 37 percent of rheumatoid arthritis patients, and cheese affected 24 percent. As this study demonstrated, dairy products such as milk, cheese and butter can definitely cause flare-ups of rheumatoid arthritis in some people. If dairy foods aggravate your arthritis, you need to read food labels to make sure that dairy products are not used in any prepared foods you're eating.

SIDESTEP CORN AND OTHER GRAINS. Corn, wheat, oats and rye aggravate rheumatoid arthritis in some people. Avoiding them is difficult because they're in so many foods— and you'll be missing out on fiber and important nutrients if you try a grain-free menu. But if they're causing the inflammation problem, you may be able to avoid them and, with a doctor's guidance, fill out your menu with other high-fiber foods and supplements to make up for the fiber and nutrients you might be missing.

LINE UP OTHER SUSPECTS. A wide variety of foods has been reported to aggravate rheumatoid arthritis in some people, including citrus foods such as oranges, grapefruit and lemons, eggs, refined sugar, peanuts or certain beverages such as coffee. One way to find out if you're allergic to any one of these foods is to drop it from your menu for a few weeks and then see what happens.

Cut the Fat, Slash the Pain

For anyone with rheumatoid arthritis, eating fat-filled foods may lead to painful consequences. Animal fats in meats, dairy products and shellfish produce hormonelike substances called prostaglandins, which are highly inflammatory.

"People can experience dramatic improvements in their symptoms when they cut back on their consumption of high-fat foods such as dairy products and red meats," says Dr. Pisetsky.

Across-the-board fat reduction combined with exercise can significantly reduce rheumatoid arthritis symptoms, according to a study conducted by Edward H. Krick, M.D., of Loma Linda University in California. Dr. Krick selected 46 people who suffered from rheumatoid arthritis and then placed half the group on a program of exercise and stress reduction. The other half was on the same program plus a very low fat diet (10 percent of total calories). After 12 weeks the low-fat group was significantly better off than the high-fat group in regard to the number of tender and swollen joints.

While you probably won't be able to reduce the fat in your diet to 10 percent of calories—that's extremely low—any reduction can help. And of course when you eat low-fat, you'll get the benefits of weight loss as well.

Put Your Diet to the Test

A growing body of evidence suggests that many common foods contain allergens, substances that trigger allergic reactions that worsen the severity of arthritis symptoms such as inflammation and stiffness. But which foods contain the allergens that are causing your problems?

To find out, the usual approach is to go on an elimination diet—a doctor-supervised program in which you're put on a total or near-total fast for several days. Ordinary foods are then added back to the diet one at a time to determine which ones make your arthritis worse. If symptoms arise following the reintroduction of a specific food, you've nabbed the culprit.

Even after you've started an elimination diet, however, it can take weeks to identify the aggravating food. Also, arthritis symptoms are sometimes slow to develop after a food is reintroduced. And of course you can't eliminate all foods at the beginning of the diet, or you'd run the risk of malnutrition.

You shouldn't try any drastic dietary manipulations without consulting a physician, advises David S. Pisetsky, M.D., PhD., medical adviser to the Arthritis Foundation. But you can try a safe, modified version of

But there is one type of fat that you don't want to cut from your diet—the omega-3 fatty acids found in abundance in the oil of cold-water fish. Omega-3's are thought to work on rheumatoid arthritis by reducing the body's production of inflammatory substances, according to Joel M. Kremer, M.D., professor of medicine and head of the Division of Rheumatology at Albany Medical College in New York. His research has shown that a diet high in omega-3 fatty acids can bring a modest reduction in inflammation.

---

the elimination diet to deduce if something in your diet is triggering your arthritis flare-ups. Here's how.

• Record your body's signals, says Dr. Pisetsky. He suggests that you write down everything you eat. After you've done this a few times, you'll be able to compare lists and see what might have led to other flare-ups. Start a list of likely suspects.

• When you've established that a certain food looks like a prime suspect, stop eating it for about a week to get it out of your system. If you feel better, you know you're getting warm. Then try the food again and see if your symptoms worsen. Repeat this test twice. If your symptoms get worse each time, you can be sure you've made a connection.

• If you've identified the aggravating food as something you don't eat often, you can probably avoid eating it and never know the difference. But if it's a very common or essential part of a balanced diet, such as a dairy product, a meat, a grain or a fruit or vegetable, see a doctor or nutritionist before you quit cold turkey. Don't give up a food unless you're sure another source will give you the nutrients provided by that food.

In one 24-week study of 49 people with rheumatoid arthritis, Dr. Kremer found that those who received high doses of fish oil had significantly less tenderness than those who didn't have any fish oil.

A Week of Vegetarian Menus

Want to try de-meating your meals? This example of a meatless menu plan features meals that are tasty, easy to prepare and rich in nutrients. It's easy to see

DAY 1

BREAKFAST

Grapefruit sections
Raisin bran cereal with low-fat or skim milk

LUNCH

Cheese ravioli with marinara sauce and
    Parmesan cheese
Tossed green salad with chick-peas, carrots and
    light dressing
Italian bread
Fresh fruit salad

DINNER

Minestrone soup
Steamed snow peas
Boston lettuce salad with low-fat blue cheese
    dressing
Whole-wheat roll
Almond cookies

SNACK

Rice cakes
All-fruit preserves

Eight to ten ounces of sardines, salmon or tuna contain about the same levels of omega-3 fatty acids used in Dr. Kremer's studies. Other fish high in omega-3's are mackerel, herring, whitefish, anchovies and bluefish.

how foods can be combined and varied to make up a total meal plan that could help relieve your arthritis symptoms.

DAY 2

BREAKFAST

> Pineapple-banana shake
> Toasted raisin bread
> Nonfat cream cheese

LUNCH

> Split pea soup with toasted croutons
> Cold rice salad with pimento and pine nuts
> Grapes

DINNER

> Penne pasta with steamed vegetables, chopped
>   olives and mozzarella cheese
> Grilled eggplant slices
> Romaine salad with chick-peas and low-fat
>   Thousand Island dressing

SNACK

> Baked apple with caramel sauce
> Hot chocolate made with low-fat milk

(continued)

Got Gout? Try These Tips

Back in the days when royalty ate roast boar while peas-
ants dined on bread and potatoes, gout was the curse of the
upper class.

Now we know why. First of all, obesity makes people
more susceptible to gout. Also, their diets were high in the
compounds known as purines—chemicals that the body

A Week of Vegetarian Menus—Continued

DAY 3

BREAKFAST

> Orange juice
> Apple pancakes with maple syrup

LUNCH

> Macaroni and cheese with chopped tomatoes
>   and zucchini
> Bitter greens with tangy dressing
> Melon balls

DINNER

> Grilled vegetable patties with lettuce and sliced
>   tomatoes on a whole-wheat bun
> Baked navy beans
> Cinnamon graham crackers
> Skim milk

SNACK

> Raisins and lightly smoked almonds

converts to uric acid, which is the substance that causes gout attacks.

Today, all of us have access to purine-rich foods. "Usually, these foods won't cause a gout attack by themselves," observes Christopher M. Wise, M.D., associate professor of internal medicine in the Division of Rheumatology at Virginia Commonwealth University of the Medical College of Virginia in Richmond. He says that certain people are "genetically pre-

---

DAY 4

BREAKFAST

Oatmeal with low-fat or skim milk
Strawberries

LUNCH

Noodle soup
Melba toast
Low-fat Monterey Jack cheese
Nonfat chocolate pudding

DINNER

Vermicelli with chunky vegetables
Escarole and red onion salad with balsamic
    vinegar
Italian bread rubbed with garlic and drizzled with
    olive oil
Steamed asparagus
Sliced kiwifruit and oranges drizzled with honey

SNACK

Plain popcorn

(continued)

disposed" to get arthritis—that is, they have an inherited gene that makes them more vulnerable to purines than others. "But if you carry that gene, and your diet is very high in purine-rich foods, that could be enough to raise your body's uric acid levels to trigger a gout attack. And if you continue eating those foods, the likelihood of future attacks will be very high," he says.

Although drugs can keep gout under control, doctors say

A Week of Vegetarian Menus—Continued

DAY 5

BREAKFAST

Peach nectar
Scrambled egg substitute with peppers
and onions

LUNCH

Pita stuffed with nonfat cream cheese,
shredded carrots and chives
Hot couscous with lentils, tomatoes and
Parmesan cheese
Celery sticks
Pineapple nonfat yogurt
Apple juice

DINNER

Vegetable lasagna
Steamed snow peas
Raw spinach with low-fat Oriental soy dressing

SNACK

Low-fat Swiss cheese and oat crackers
Pears

that even medication is more effective if gout-prone people watch their diets. Here are the strategies.

PASS ON PURINES. These compounds are found in many different types of foods, but most have insignificant amounts. You can avoid the worst offenders, including organ meats such as liver and kidneys and foods that contain gravies and meat extracts. Unfortunately, some fish that are very healthful in other respects—including those high omega-3 sources such as

---

DAY 6

BREAKFAST

Cranberry juice
Vidalia onion omelet
Toasted bagel
Nonfat cream cheese

LUNCH

Baked potato
Hearty lentil chili
Mixed green salad with low-fat Dijon dressing
Mixed dried fruit

DINNER

Baked winter squash stuffed with wild rice
Steamed green beans with sesame seeds
Tossed green salad with low-fat Oriental
    soy dressing
Raspberry fruit-and-yogurt bar

SNACK

Dried apple rings

(continued)

anchovies, herring and mackerel—also contain purines. It's also wise to avoid high-purine shellfish such as shrimp, scallops, crab, lobster and oysters.

Some vegetables have purines, though not as much as the worst offenders. The ones to watch out for include spinach, asparagus and mushrooms. People with gout should also steer clear of peas, kidney beans, lentils and lima beans.

DRINK LOTS OF WATER. Dr. Pisetsky recommends that you keep sipping water throughout the day. The extra fluid helps flush uric acid out of the body before it can crystallize.

A Week of Vegetarian Menus—Continued

DAY 7

BREAKFAST

French toast
Low-fat milk
Blueberries

LUNCH

Cheese pizza
Roasted red peppers and blanched green
   beans with balsamic vinegar
Nonfat yogurt with raisins, cinnamon
   and honey

DINNER

Vegetable kabobs
Baked sweet potato
Couscous with grated orange peel
Banana fruit shake

SNACK

Ice milk with chopped nuts and
   pineapple topping

SHED POUNDS—BUT NOT TOO QUICKLY. If you're overweight and gout-prone, you should back off on high-fat foods. But the goal is to lose weight gradually. Doctors advise against a starvation-type diet that produces very rapid weight loss.

In fact, a crash diet can aggravate gout rather than help it. "Sudden, rapid burning of body fat can produce high uric acid levels in some people," says Dr. Wise.

TEND TOWARD TEETOTALING. Gout sufferers should drink alcohol in very small amounts, if at all, says Dr. Wise. That's because alcohol tends to make uric acid levels rise. In addition, beverages such as wine and beer have a high purine content.

The Ultimate Pain-Away Plan

Many rheumatologists and researchers recommend a vegetarian diet. They've found that some people who switch to a vegetarian diet can sustain the benefits that come from fasting even though they start eating again. The difference is that they don't eat everything—just certain vegetarian-type foods.

To see if people on a vegetarian diet would be as pain-free as those who fasted, researchers from the University of Oslo in Norway and the National Hospital in Oslo set up an experiment involving 53 people, all of whom had arthritis. Dividing the participants into two groups, researchers placed one group on a fast and allowed the other group to eat its usual diet.

During an initial seven- to ten-day fast, participants consumed only herbal teas, garlic, vegetable broth, water and various vegetable juices. After that, researchers gradually introduced the components of a vegetarian diet: noncitrus fruits, vegetables, gluten-free whole grains and legumes. But the participants continued to abstain from any foods that contained meat, fish, eggs, dairy products, gluten (a component found in wheat), refined sugar, salt, spices, preservatives and citrus fruits.

One month from the beginning of the study, people who

had started by fasting and then switched to a vegetarian diet reported significant reductions in their arthritis symptoms. They had a decrease in the number of tender joints, less morning stiffness and pain and considerably more grip strength.

After three to five months the experimental group was allowed to gradually begin eating foods containing gluten, such as bread and wheat products, along with milk and other dairy products. The participants maintained this diet for another eight to ten months.

Finally, after a total of 13 months, researchers compared the group that was now on a full vegetarian diet with the

A Carnivore's Guide to Going Vegetarian

If you switch to a vegetarian diet, you might be concerned about getting all of the nutrients you need. But you don't have to worry as long as you get plenty of variety—and include milk and eggs (if you're not allergic to them) as well as vegetables in your diet.

It's the strict vegetarian diets—the kind that allow no fish, dairy products or eggs—that need to be carefully supervised to make sure that you get all the nutrients you need. "When you eliminate meats and dairy products, you eliminate the best sources of certain nutrients," says Jeffrey R. Lisse, M.D., associate professor of medicine and director of the Division of Rheumatology at the University of Texas Medical Branch at the University of Texas Medical School at Galveston.

But with some planning, you can make up all or most of the nutrients that are found in meats. Here are some guidelines to keep in mind.

• If you omit all animal products from your diet, you may lack protein. So make sure your diet focuses

group that had not changed its diet at all. The conclusions were decisive. The symptoms of the group that had stuck to an "ordinary" diet either stayed the same or got worse. But the experimental group reported continued improvement in their symptoms even when they switched over to a vegetarian diet.

In other words, the benefits of fasting persisted as long as those people continued with their individualized vegetarian diets.

Although a vegetarian diet might not be for everyone, this study shows that it might make a dramatic difference for some people who have very painful symptoms.

---

on protein-rich plant foods, such as legumes (beans and peas) and nuts.

• If you give up meat, you're also giving up the iron, zinc and vitamins that meat provides. You can get more of these vital nutrients by eating legumes, tofu, whole grains, prunes, raisins, spinach, nuts and seeds, fortified cereals and green, leafy vegetables.

• Anyone who cuts out dairy products is giving up the richest source of calcium. This can increase your risk of osteoporosis as well as contribute to further joint damage. You can get a calcium boost from dark green, leafy vegetables, tofu, legumes and calcium-fortified orange juice. You may also want to take supplements.

• Vitamin B_{12}, an essential nutrient, is found exclusively in animal foods. If you eliminate eggs, dairy products and meats, you'll have to rely on fortified cereals or supplements to get your daily dose. But if you give up only meat—and not eggs or dairy foods—you'll be more likely to get the B_{12} you need.

The Benefits of Going Meatless

Why does a vegetarian diet sometimes take the fire out of inflammation?

Researchers have a few theories. For one thing, people tend to be allergic to fewer substances in vegetables than in meat and dairy products.

Vegetables may also provide benefits because of what they don't contain. "A vegetarian diet is usually low in calories and fat," says Dr. Pisetsky. "We don't know why, but a low-calorie, low-fat diet seems to somehow improve the function of the immune system in some people, and that results in less inflammation and other symptoms."

For most people, making the transition from omnivore to herbivore doesn't really require a major lifestyle adjustment. And it doesn't mean that you have to start eating weird foods that you've never heard of before. Today you can go meatless and still enjoy meals that are flavorful, filling and satisfying.

Besides, vegetarianism doesn't necessarily have to be an all-or-nothing affair. "Most arthritis patients probably don't need to become complete vegetarians to enjoy the benefits that vegetarianism often provides," says Dr. Pisetsky. "Many people benefit simply by incorporating elements of vegetarianism. They cut back somewhat on their red meat or dairy consumption while increasing their fruits and vegetables. Or, if they're sensitive to red meat, they replace it with poultry and fish."

Back Pain
Take the Low-Fat Road

IF YOUR BACK HURTS as you reach for the crisper drawer in the fridge, you're probably not keeping the right things in it. Recent research suggests that fatty foods may be at the root of your back pain.

Studies of the arteries of 86 average-weight men showed that the greater the plaque deposits, the greater the degeneration of spinal disks. Other studies by the same team have also shown an association between narrowed or missing arteries and lower-back pain. Until now, few researchers have looked at blood flow to the spine because the standard methods of investigating that area don't show the blood vessels.

The main focus in these studies was the abdominal aorta, the major blood pathway to the lumbar spine and often one of the first spots where plaque builds up. "Compromised blood supply affects disks, muscles, nerve roots and other structures in the lower spine and causes degeneration as it does in any other organ suffering from diminished blood supply," says Leena I. Kauppila, M.D., study leader and visiting researcher in the orthopedic department at Harvard Medical School.

Exercise may help small, new vessels develop, "but probably will never compensate completely," she says.

That means your best strategy is prevention. "To minimize further disk degeneration, people with lower-back symptoms and/or premature disk degeneration without obvious cause ought to think about their diets," Dr. Kauppila says. And that means the usual health-smart, low-fat fare. Of course, there are many reasons for lower-back symptoms. Those of a few days' duration are probably from some other cause. Back pain with leg pain that doesn't go away in a day or two and extreme weakness in an extremity are good reasons to call your doctor right away.

···

Bladder Infections
An Infection-Fighting "Cocktail"

YOU MAY HAVE HEARD about this for-women-only folk remedy. And now there's a scientific study that validates it: Women fighting bladder infections with cranberry juice cocktail may be doing the right thing.

When 72 postmenopausal women downed ten ounces of the juice per day for six months, they were 58 percent less likely to develop urinary tract infections than women who drank a look-alike, noncranberry juice with the same amount of vitamin C. The juice seemed to have an even more powerful effect on infections already in progress. Cranberry juice drinkers were only a quarter as likely to have their infections continue, compared with women who were drinking the placebo.

Earlier theories suggested that vitamin C was the active compound. Vitamin C was believed to stifle the infections by acidifying the urine. But more recent evidence suggests something different, says study leader Jerry Avorn, M.D., associate professor of medicine at Harvard Medical School. "There's a substance in cranberries that may prevent the adhesiveness of bacteria to the bladder wall. We don't know if that's what was going on in our study, but it's a pretty interesting possibility," he says.

"People who have been drinking this can now say that they were right," he says. "But this doesn't mean that cranberries can replace antibiotics. If you're having symptoms of an infection, you still need to see your doctor."

Older women, like those in this study, have a high prevalence of these infections, yet don't usually have the raging symptoms—a burning feeling during urination and the need to urinate frequently—that are more common among the younger set. So researchers are hesitant to say just yet what cranberry juice might mean to premenopausal women. For now, says Dr. Avorn, "If women find that cranberry juice works for them, that's great. But if you have symptoms, the right thing to do is seek medical attention.

....

Blood Pressure
Send It South with Beans and Bananas

IF YOU HAVE HIGH BLOOD PRESSURE (defined as a reading of 140/90 and above), you want powerful medicine to control it. And—as study after study has shown—diet is powerful medicine. It can't always replace pills and other medical means when blood pressure is elevated, but it often does. And it can frequently either boost the effect of medication or allow for a lower dose. More good news: Those who are helped the most by good eating are the ones who most need help. The higher your blood pressure, the more it is likely to fall if you use your head when you fill your belly.

Diet therapy to reduce high blood pressure calls for the following:

- An eating plan geared to weight control. For those people who are overweight, a low-fat diet (made up of less than 20 percent of calories), high in unrefined complex carbohydrates is ideal.
- Limiting sodium intake to 2,400 milligrams a day (the amount in a level teaspoon of table salt). Discuss with your physician whether it would be wise to limit your sodium intake even more.

- Including in your diet a variety of fruits and vegetables that together provide at least 3,500 milligrams of potassium a day.
- Getting your Daily Value (DV) for magnesium (400 milligrams) and calcium (1,000 milligrams).

Are You Sodium-Sensitive?

Being sodium-sensitive means that your blood pressure rises in reaction to increased sodium intake. "All people are, more or less, sodium-sensitive. And there is no sharp break between those who are more sensitive and those who are less,"

Lick Your Taste for Salt

If salt seems like something that your taste buds just can't do without, consider this: Salt may actually hide flavor. And if you're absolutely convinced that you're addicted to salt, you must know this: Tastes change.

"People who've cut down on salt often find months after that salty food tastes terrible," says Harvey B. Simon, M.D., professor of preventive cardiology at Harvard Medical School and a founding member of the Harvard Cardiovascular Health Center.

"After you shake the habit and discover the real taste of food, you don't want the taste covered up by salt. In fact, you feel terribly thirsty after eating salty food, and it's a very uncomfortable feeling."

Of course, you're wondering how to get to this wonderfully unsalted state of mind. Dr. Simon advises that you trick your taste buds by changing very gradually. "Begin by substituting low-sodium foods for the highly salted variety. They may seem bland at first, but in a little while, you'll actually start to like them. And besides the salt, you'll begin tasting the food.

says Norman Kaplan, M.D., professor of internal medicine in the hypertension division at the University of Texas Southwestern Medical School in Dallas. "Some people are exquisitely sensitive. If they touch salt, their blood pressure goes way up. For a few others, their intake hardly seems to matter."

About half of people with high blood pressure fit into the category of highly sodium-sensitive. For many of these people, sodium restriction is definitely a good idea. Among those people who are not sodium-sensitive, restricting salt too much —to less than half a teaspoon a day—also may raise their blood pressure. So if you happen to be sodium-sensitive, what should you do?

"Next, wean yourself from the saltshaker. Measuring the amount of salt you're sprinkling over food will help you measure your progress, and it may surprise you to see just how much you've been adding.

"At the same time, begin eliminating the salt from your cooking. Look upon all this as a great opportunity to experiment with new flavors and seasonings. Your taste buds will love you," says Dr. Simon.

Some flavors may be particularly effective substitutes. "Sour flavors can mimic a salty flavor," says Beverly Cowart, Ph.D., clinic director at the Monell Chemical Senses Center in Philadelphia. "So some people tend to confuse salty with sour. Citric acid, sometimes called 'sour salt' and a component of lemon juice, is one example.

"There are some similarities in how salty and sour are perceived by the tongue. So some people may find lemon juice or vinegar to be acceptable alternatives to salt, providing a similar flavor," she says. So, salt lovers, be brave. Cutting back on salt isn't deprivation but a gift to your taste buds!

The best approach is to start by making sure that you get no more sodium than your body needs. The average American consumes about 4,000 milligrams of sodium each day. That's quite a few shakes beyond the 2,400 milligrams that the National Academy of Sciences suggests as a maximum intake for just about everyone. A level teaspoon of salt contains about 2,400 milligrams of sodium, so if your current intake is 3,500 milligrams or less, you can get yourself to the adequate intake zone by getting rid of about half a teaspoon of salt each day.

The next step is to check with your doctor to see if you might benefit from further cuts in sodium intake. There's currently no standard test to determine if you're sodium-sensitive—or if your blood pressure might rise because of serious sodium restriction. But you and your doctor might be able to determine if you're sensitive to sodium through dietary trial and error. Harvey B. Simon, M.D., professor of preventive cardiology at Harvard Medical School, a founding member of the Harvard Cardiovascular Health Center and author of *Conquering Heart Disease,* suggests cutting sodium intake to 2,000 milligrams a day for six weeks. If your blood pressure goes down, that's a strong indication that you're sodium-sensitive. So if some form of sodium restriction is your objective, what's a good plan of attack?

Sidestepping the Salt Mines

There are several ways that you can cut your intake of sodium, and some are less obvious than others.

First, cut back on the saltshaker. "That's what we go after," says Dr. Kaplan. "Salt poured on food is the thing people have the most immediate control over."

Then go after the foods that Dr. Kaplan calls "salt mines"—for example, anchovies, sauerkraut, pickles and salami. "All we're talking about here is taking a few of life's pleasures away," says Dr. Kaplan. "It won't be easy for those few people who are addicted to salami. But it's usually not a major sacrifice."

The greatest salt mine of all, though, just may be potato chips. "You would need to eat ten whole potatoes to get the amount of sodium in just ten potato chips," says Dr. Simon.

The next sodium source on your list should be processed foods, because salt and other sodium compounds act as preservatives and flavor enhancers and are often used liberally in them. Not surprisingly, processed foods (which include some of the worst salt mines already mentioned) are far and away the biggest source of sodium in the American diet, perhaps accounting for more than 70 percent of our intake. (By contrast, the sodium naturally present in foods accounts for about 12 percent.) Canned foods are the worst offenders. But you can find a high sodium content in some frozen foods, baked goods and many staples at fast-food restaurants. Reading food

Label Shakeout

Uncle Sam has stepped in to bring order to the once chaotic world of food labels. Here's what those words mean.

Sodium-free. Less than 5 milligrams per serving. No need to restrict yourself, since 400 servings a day would still keep you at 2,000 milligrams of sodium.

Very low sodium. Thirty-five milligrams or less per serving. You're still in the safe zone.

Low sodium. Means 140 milligrams or less per serving. Don't get reckless. A few servings can add up in a hurry.

Reduced sodium. Three-quarters less sodium than is typical for that food. Fact is, many foods are typically high in sodium, so reducing that amount may not be as helpful as you think. Also, the container may not say simply "salt." Don't be fooled by sea salt, garlic salt, onion salt, seasoned salt or brine.

Note: If a serving size is very small—for example two tablespoons of salad dressing—then 35 to 140 milligrams can still be quite a high concentration of sodium for such a small portion.

labels is critical to finding your way past the salt mines in the supermarket.

How much of a difference does all this sodium searching really make? Well, for many people, for each teaspoon of salt they eliminate, they can expect a five-point drop in systolic (top number of your blood pressure reading) pressure and half that in diastolic (bottom number) pressure. For millions of Americans, this would be enough of a drop to eliminate the need for medications.

Pump Up the Potassium

Now we switch from what you need less of to what you need more of. "You can think of potassium as the opposite of sodium," says Dr. Simon. Just as a high sodium intake can

Potassium-Packed Foods

Power up your diet with some of these potassium-rich foods.

FOOD	POTASSIUM (mg.)
½ cup dried apricots	896
½ cup dried peaches	784
1 cup cooked plantain slices	716
1 cup plain low-fat yogurt	531
1 boiled potato, cooked in skin	515
3 ounces baked or broiled halibut	490
½ cup boiled lima beans	478
1 banana	451
1 boiled potato cooked without skin	443
1 sweet potato baked in skin	397
½ cup boiled baby lima beans	365
½ cup boiled kidney beans	355
½ cup All-Bran	340
½ cup canned kidney beans	329
½ cup winter squash, boiled, mashed	321

raise blood pressure, so too can a low potassium intake, since potassium works as a blood vessel dilator. But this doesn't mean that huge amounts of potassium are needed.

The DV for potassium is 3,500 milligrams, "but it's safe to consume substantially more than that," says Dr. Simon. The trick is getting enough potassium in your daily menu without going on the chimpanzee diet. Actually, bananas are not the highest source of potassium, which can be found in a wide assortment of fruits and vegetables. And there are some surprisingly rich sources.

One caution: If you're taking a potassium-sparing diuretic, which causes the kidneys to hoard the mineral, you should not increase your potassium intake without discussing with your doctor any changes you'd like to make.

More Depressurizing Minerals

Along with potassium, you can add calcium and magnesium to the list of minerals that may help lower your blood pressure through some unknown ways. People with high blood pressure tend to have lower consumption of all three.

Sources of Magnesium

The following foods are packed with magnesium.

FOOD	MAGNESIUM (mg.)
½ cup 100% Bran	121
½ cup All-Bran	120
2 tablespoons dried pumpkin seed kernels	92
¼ cup wheat bran	86
½ cup boiled wax beans	65
2 tablespoons toasted wheat germ	45
½ cup Bran Chex	41
6 medium oysters, steamed	40
½ cup lima beans, boiled	40
½ cup Bran Buds	40

African-Americans seem to be especially vulnerable to low calcium intake.

As with potassium, you don't necessarily need calcium and magnesium by the shovelful. Instead, you simply need to be certain you're getting the DV for these minerals.

....

Cancer Prevention
Diet Can Make a Difference

HERE'S A SHOCKER: Experts estimate that eating a poor diet is responsible for anywhere from 10 to 70 percent of all cancers. "And I think it's probably closer to 70 percent than it is to 10," says Gladys Block, Ph.D., professor of public health nutrition at the University of California at Berkeley and an expert on nutrition and cancer.

That's where *Prevention* magazine's Anti-Cancer Eating Plan comes in. Of course, regular exercise, smoking cessation and appropriate screenings, such as Pap tests and prostate exams, are also crucial.

That said, the right diet can go a long way to bolster your resistance.

Its core features are:

• Cutting fat intake to less than 20 percent of total calories and saturated fat intake to less than 10 grams per day.

• Focusing on a plant-based diet rich in a diverse assortment of vegetables, fruits, grains and beans, which are naturally low-fat and high-fiber and are key sources of important vitamins and other food factors linked to lower cancer risk. Ideally, the daily diet should include at least 9 servings of fruits and vegetables and from 6 to 11 servings of whole-grain breads, cereals, pastas, brown rice and legumes.

- Restricting meat.
- Including at least one serving a day of tofu or other soy food.
- Eating fish several times a week.

Be Adventurous with Veggies

So why is diversity in plant-based foods so important? First, despite the flurry of research on the cancer-preventing properties of specific foods such as broccoli, garlic and carrots, experts cannot yet say which, if any, is the best. Indeed, they suspect that different foods and nutrients work together as a team to combat cancer. Second, diversity in your diet can also keep your palate satisfied, so you're less likely to resort to your old ways of eating.

High intakes of fruits and vegetables have been associated with lower risks of just about every type of cancer, from breast, bladder, lung and prostate to stomach, cervical and ovarian. In many studies people who loaded their plates with fruits and vegetables cut their risk of cancers by half—or more—compared with those who ate the fewest fruits and veggies.

While experts haven't determined the optimum "dose" of produce to prevent cancer, the research so far suggests that "there's no such thing as too much when it comes to fruits and vegetables," says Dr. Block.

For now, aim for nine (or more) servings, making sure that you choose at least one serving from each of the following categories: citrus fruits, cruciferous vegetables (such as broccoli, cauliflower or cabbage), dark green, leafy vegetables (such as spinach or romaine lettuce) and yellow-orange fruits and vegetables.

It seems that the treasures of our gardens and groves pack a triple threat against carcinogens: Vegetables and fruits are potent sources of antioxidants, which may protect genetic materials from damage from cancer-causing agents, thus halting the earliest processes that lead to cancer. Fruits and vegetables are rich in soluble fiber, which may help harmful substances to be excreted in the stool. And they're chock-full of literally thousands of compounds—called phytochemicals—many of which have been shown in test-tube studies to stunt the growth of cancer cells. (See "Cancer-Phyting Foods.")

Because many phytochemicals have yet to be isolated and tested, researchers refrain from recommending one class or food source over another. Your best bet is to eat a variety, Dr. Block says.

Cancer and Fat: Here's the Skinny

Breast cancer. Colorectal cancer. Prostate cancer. Pancreatic and endometrial cancer. Dietary fat has been linked to all of these and more—even lung cancer in nonsmokers.

Saturated fat, the type found in meats, cheeses, egg yolks, butter and other whole-milk dairy products, seems to be particularly dangerous. In a recent three-year review of about 1,000 women's diets, it was found that women who ate a mere ten grams (the amount in one cheeseburger with fixings) of saturated fat per day had a 20 percent higher risk of ovarian cancer than women at lower consumption levels. But even an excess of the polyunsaturated fats in vegetable oils and margarine may contribute to your cancer risk.

Researchers aren't quite sure how eating fatty foods affects your cancer risk, but they have a couple of theories. Too many of those cheeseburgers may lead to colon cancer by stimulating the production of excess acids that irritate the lining of the colon. High intake of fatty foods may also increase the level of estrogen in the blood, high levels of which have been associated with breast cancer.

Prevention magazine's Anti-Cancer Eating Plan recommendation of less than 20 percent of calories from fat is substantially lower than the 40 percent consumed by most Americans and the 30 percent suggested by the National Cancer Institute. If you're a woman who eats about 1,800 calories a day, your maximum fat budget is 39 grams; men who take in 2,600 calories a day should limit their fat intake to 56 grams.

Cancer-Phyting Foods

Here is a list of the 14 general classes of phyto-chemicals, as well as the foods they're found in, that research has identified as possible cancer fighters. Experts emphasize that you get these phytochemicals when you eat a mixture of vegetables and fruits.

- Carotenoids—Cruciferous vegetables such as broccoli, cabbage, brussels sprouts, cauliflower and bok choy; greens, carrots, tomatoes, pumpkin, winter squash, melon, citrus fruits
- Coumarins—Parsley, parsnips, cucumbers
- Flavonoids—Soybeans (including soy-based foods such as tofu and tempeh); eggplant, flax
- Glucarates—Whole grains, cruciferous vegetables, citrus fruits, tomatoes, eggplant, peppers
- Indoles—Cruciferous vegetables
- Isothiocyanates—Cruciferous vegetables
- Lignins—Soybeans and soy products, flaxseed
- Monoterpenes—Garlic, cruciferous vegetables, citrus fruits, parsley, carrots, celery, cucumbers, parsnips, squash, tomatoes, eggplant, peppers, fennel
- Phenolic acids—Cruciferous vegetables, greens, carrots, celery, parsley, parsnips, tomatoes, eggplant, peppers, cucumbers, pumpkin, squash, melon, soybeans, citrus fruits
- Phthalides—Carrots, celery, parsley, parsnips, fennel
- Phytates—Soybeans and soy products, whole grains
- Polyacetylenes—Fennel, celery, parsley, carrots
- Sulfides—Garlic, cruciferous vegetables, onions
- Triterpenes—Garlic, soybeans, whole grains, cruciferous vegetables, celery, carrots, tomatoes, cucumbers, squash, eggplant, peppers

Go with the Grain

Along with the soluble fiber that you get from the vegetables you eat, you need insoluble fiber, the kind found in whole grains such as wheat and oat bran. That type of fiber has been found to be extremely effective in lowering risk of colon cancer because, scientists believe, it helps dilute potentially harmful bile acids and carry them out of the body in the stool.

Hints for Hard-Core Carnivores

There are ways to make meatless meals seem, well, not meatless. "The right tricks can help you mimic the hearty, homey feeling you get from meat-based dishes," says Linda Rosensweig, author of the cookbook *New Vegetarian Cuisine*. Here are some of her secrets.

• Make a rich, beef broth–like base for veggie soups and stews. Sauté vegetables (such as onions, green and red peppers and mushrooms) in a frying pan lightly sprayed with oil and place them in a separate dish. Then add vegetable broth (either canned or homemade) to the pan, scraping the browned bits from the bottom.

• Choose rib-sticking tomato- and legume-based dishes. "Heavy tomato sauces for pasta, vegetarian chili and entrées like lentil soup are so hearty you won't miss the meat," Rosensweig says.

• Use mushrooms instead of meat. Giant portobello mushrooms taste great grilled and have a chewy, substantial texture. Simply remove the stems, brush the caps lightly with oil and grill until crispy. Slice and mix with salad greens and other garden veggies for a meatless chef salad.

Insoluble fiber may also help rid your body of cancer-causing agents that threaten the breast, prostate and pancreas. Whole-grain foods, and especially legumes, are also good sources of folate. Low levels of this B vitamin have been linked to breast cancer and a condition known as cervical dysplasia, a precursor to cervical cancer.

Research hasn't yet identified the optimum ratio of soluble to insoluble fiber. But your 9 daily fruits and vegetables plus

....

• Check your grocery store's freezer or refrigerated deli-meat section for fast-food fare, some made with a mixture of grains and seeds, others tofu-based. (Be sure to read labels, though—some weigh in heavy when it comes to fat.) Serve them up on whole-wheat rolls with all the accoutrements, and your taste buds won't know the difference!

• Try tofu or tempeh. Crumble firm, low-fat tofu or tempeh (another soybean-based product) into pasta sauces, chilies and casseroles. (Make sure the tofu or tempeh you buy says "low-fat" on the label. The regular versions are rather high in fat.) Fold into a corn or nonfat flour tortilla with steamed veggies, spoon on some spicy salsa, and you have a tasty cancer-fighting fajita. *Qué sabrosa!*

• Get hooked on firm-fleshed fish. Hot off the barbie, tuna, mako shark, swordfish or salmon steaks give even the most stalwart carnivore something to sink his teeth into. You can even baste these meatier fine-finned friends with your favorite spicy barbecue sauce or low-sodium steak sauce if you'd like. (But keep the heavy sauces off the salmon, Rosensweig says—they'll overwhelm its more delicate flavor.)

the 6 to 11 servings of grains will put you over the top when it comes to the 30 grams of total fiber recommended to prevent most cancers. For reference, that's more than twice what the average American eats. If it's substantially more than what you're eating now, increase your intake gradually so you'll be less likely to have gastrointestinal discomfort.

Soy: Don't Knock It 'til You've Tried It

Soybeans and soy-based foods such as tofu, tempeh and soy milk contain a phytochemical known as genistein that has

MEGA-VEGETARIAN LASAGNA

ৎ

A flavorful cancer fighter, this tasty dish is a great source of vitamins A and C, folate, potassium, magnesium and iron.

3 medium sweet potatoes
1 pound fresh spinach, cleaned and trimmed
9 ounces firm tofu
1 cup nonfat ricotta cheese
1 teaspoon dried oregano
½ teaspoon dried basil
¼ cup parsley
1 large or 2 small cloves fresh garlic, pressed or minced
1 jar (32 ounces) low-fat spaghetti sauce
8 ounces shredded nonfat mozzarella cheese
3 tablespoons wheat germ

Peel and thinly slice the sweet potatoes; set aside. Lightly steam the spinach; drain and set aside.

For the filling, drain the tofu slightly, but don't squeeze out the water. Place with the ricotta in the container of a blender or food processor and blend until

proved in test-tube studies to stymie the growth of breast cancer cells and precancerous cells in the prostate gland. A soy diet may also decrease your chances of getting breast cancer by restraining the surges of estrogen that come during a menstrual cycle—and that have been fingered as a cause of breast cancer—suggests a recent study. What's more, the rates of breast cancer and prostate cancer are considerably lower in cultures that include soy dishes in their diets.

Two caveats: Stick to low-fat (1 percent fat) tofu, tempeh and soy milk. Regular versions of these products get anywhere from 30 to over 50 percent of their calories from fat. And, the

smooth. Transfer to a bowl and add the oregano, basil, parsley and garlic, mixing well.

To assemble the lasagna, spread a thin layer of the sauce in the bottom of a 9″ × 13″ baking pan. Cover with a layer of sweet potato slices (about one-third of the veggies). Spread half the filling over the sweet potatoes. Cover with one-third of the remaining sauce and sprinkle with half the mozzarella. Layer with the spinach. Layer with another third of the sweet potatoes and the remaining filling. Cover with another third of the sauce and the remaining mozzarella. Layer with the rest of the sweet potatoes, cover with the remaining sauce and sprinkle with the wheat germ.

Bake for 45 minutes at 375°. Let stand for 10 minutes before serving.

MAKES 6 SERVINGS

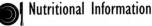 ## Nutritional Information

Per serving: 297 calories, 4.6 g. fat (14% of calories), 0 mg. cholesterol, 426 milligrams sodium, 6.6 g. dietary fiber.

Sample Cancer-Shielding Menu

Cancer-proofing your body doesn't have to deprive your taste buds. Check out the sample menu below.

FOOD	TOTAL FAT (g.)
BREAKFAST	
1 cup bran flakes	0
1 cup bran flakes with ½ cup 1% low-fat milk	1
½ banana, sliced*	0
¾ cup orange juice	0
LUNCH	
STIR-FRY VEGGIE PLATE	
2 cups veggies	1
2 teaspoons olive oil	9
1 cup brown rice	2
1 cup black bean soup*	2
SNACK	
Large apple	0
15 almonds*	12.5
DINNER	
Mega-vegetarian Lasagna (see page 82)*	4.6
½ (8-ounce) Italian bread shell*	3
1 cup nonfat frozen yogurt	0
TOTAL	**35.1**

NOTE: Also contains 1,771 calories (18% of calories from fat), 6 servings of grains/legumes (including 1 serving of soy food), 9 servings of fruits and vegetables.

*For men, double the portions of these foods, except the almonds (men can have 24). You'll get 2,520 calories with 52.2 g. fat (19% of calories), 8 servings of grains/legumes (including 2 servings of soy food), 12 servings of fruits and vegetables.

health benefits of soy don't apply to soy sauce! For more information about soy, see "Heart and Soy" on page 285.

The "Fat" That Helps Clobber Cancer
....

Fish fats—known as omega-3 fatty acids—seem to have the opposite effect on cancer risk from other types of fat. Studies have suggested that increasing the amount of omega-3's in the diet (while decreasing other types of fat) can lower the incidence of breast cancer tumors. And seafood is a great source of selenium, a mineral that at insufficient intake levels may be associated with prostate and pancreatic cancer.

Some of the best sources of omega-3's are herring, salmon, sardines, mackerel, swordfish, whitefish and Pacific oysters.

....

Carpal Tunnel Syndrome
A Nutritional Twist for a Painful Wrist

WHEN YOU HAVE carpal tunnel syndrome (CTS), your median nerve, one of three that supplies the hand, is "pinched." As a result, the thumb and middle three fingers tingle, feel numb and hurt. Your wrist and forearm might also be painful. The most common cause of CTS is a mechanical one—the result of chronic, repetitive motion and overuse of the hands or wrists—so you're a candidate if you are a typist, computer operator, butcher, carpenter or store cashier. Tissues surrounding the median nerve become irritated and swollen and impinge upon it.

The median nerve can also be affected by several non-mechanical conditions. For example, when the immune system is not functioning properly, as occurs in people with rheumatoid arthritis, tendons and ligaments surrounding the nerve swell and compress it. Low thyroid function causes retention of fluid, engorging the structures that surround the median nerve. The nerve itself may become irritated in people with diabetes and in people undergoing kidney dialysis. (CTS may also surface suddenly during pregnancy and often disappears soon after delivery.)

Treatment of CTS depends on its cause. If it's caused by mechanical irritation from repetitive movement, you have to stop or change that movement, at least until the symptoms subside. You may be given a temporary splint or have your painful wrist injected with steroids to reduce inflammation and swelling. If the ligaments entrapping the nerve are thick and swollen, the nerve may have to be surgically released. This can now be done by new endoscopic techniques that are much simpler than the more extensive "open" operation.

You May Benefit from Bs

If your CTS is caused by an underactive thyroid gland, replacing the missing thyroid hormone will clear the symptoms. Most other nonmechanical causes respond to dietary measures. Taking 150 milligrams of supplemental vitamin B_6 daily for about four months (the Daily Value, or DV, is 2 milligrams) will raise your pain threshold and ease your symptoms. It does not, however, affect the underlying process, which usually runs its course during that time. Although the supplemental B_6 doesn't affect the function of the involved median nerve as measured in objective tests, it can still help make you feel better—and that's what really counts. Adding 100 micrograms of supplemental B_{12} daily by mouth (its DV is 6 micrograms) may help too, but unlike B_6, its effectiveness has not been confirmed. So if you have CTS from diabetes or other nonmechanical factors, try vitamin therapy before opting for splinting and surgery.

Why supplements and not just lots of B_6 and B_{12} in your diet? Because the amounts of these vitamins present in food is not great enough to control the pain of CTS. But if for some reason you're averse to taking supplements, the richest natural sources of vitamin B_6 are liver, oatmeal, bananas, rice bran, wheat germ, chicken, fish and sunflower seeds, and there is some in avocados and meat, too. You can obtain lots of B_{12} in organ meats such as liver as well as fish, shellfish, muscle meats, eggs and cheese.

So if you wake up one morning with a painful hand and wrist, and the pain continues for days, see your doctor. If the diagnosis is CTS, try 150 milligrams of B_6 a day, with or without supplemental B_{12}, before submitting to a cast, injections or surgery of any kind. This is especially important to remember if you have diabetes or do not use your hands every day in hours of repetitive functions. Anti-inflammatory drugs such as ibuprofen will also provide at least temporary relief. Remember, however, that doses of vitamin B_6 higher than the recommended 150 milligrams per day may have a toxic effect on the nerves, causing generalized body pain. If you're pregnant, check with your doctor before taking these (or any) vitamin supplements in high doses.

Cholesterol Control
An Artery De-gunking Plan

IF YOU'RE READY TO CLOBBER high cholesterol—that's any reading of over 200 milligrams per deciliter (mg/dl)—here's the diet for you! It's a mostly vegetarian, ultra low fat eating plan that may do more than simply chop cholesterol readings, as important as that is. According to research by *Prevention* magazine adviser Dean Ornish, M.D., author of *Dr. Dean Ornish's Program for Reversing Heart Disease without Drugs or Surgery* and *Eat More, Weigh Less*, this diet may even help clear away the cholesterol that's already built up inside your arteries.

Here are the key features.

- Slashing total fat intake to 10 percent of calories, driving saturated fat, trans-fatty acids and cholesterol as low as they can go.
- Getting at least ten grams of soluble fiber a day.
- Focusing on a mostly plant-based diet rich in vegetables, fruits, grains and beans, which are naturally low in fat and high in fiber.
- Limiting foods of animal origin, which are high in saturated fat and the sole dietary source of cholesterol— that is, using only nonfat dairy products and egg whites and limiting meat to one serving of lean poultry or fish (no red meat) three times a week.
- Eating three mini-meals plus three snacks instead of three square meals a day. (For a representative day, see "Clobber Cholesterol—Deliciously" on page 90.)

Super Sources of Soluble Fiber

Getting ten grams or more of soluble fiber a day can slice elevated cholesterol levels by 5 to 10 percent, studies indicate. So feature these soluble-fiber all-stars in your menu lineup.

FOOD	SOLUBLE FIBER (g.)
⅓ cup Kellogg's Bran Buds	3
I cup cooked Quaker Oat Bran	3
½ cup cooked kidney beans	2.8
½ cup canned baked beans	2.6
I medium cooked artichoke	2.2
I cup cooked oatmeal	2
¾ cup cooked pearl barley	1.8
½ cup cooked sweet potato	1.8
I medium baked potato with skin	1.6
2 dried figs	1.5
I orange	1.4

And here's the big payoff: By holding total fat to roughly 10 percent of calories (that's 20 grams of fat for an 1,800-calorie diet), you sidestep every known booster of blood cholesterol—too much total fat, saturated fat, trans-fatty acids and dietary cholesterol. Experts estimate that for every 1 percent drop in blood cholesterol that results, your heart attack risk drops 2 percent.

Note: The American Heart Association recommends holding daily fat intake to under 30 percent of total calories, but some heart experts now say that keeping fat at 20 percent and under is best for optimal health. If you want to take your fat consumption below 20 percent, however, you should first check with your doctor.

But there's a second payoff: On this plant-based diet, you naturally munch lots of soluble fiber, a proven choles-

PRONTO PINTO CHIPS

In minutes you can whip up this tempting heart-smart snack. It's low in fat but high in soluble fiber and satisfaction!

½ cup canned pinto beans, rinsed and drained
2 tablespoons chunky salsa
2 tablespoons fat-free sour cream
22 baked tortilla chips

In small dish, mash the beans with a fork; mix in the salsa and sour cream. Serve as dip with chips.

MAKES 1 SERVING

 Nutritional Information

Per serving: 260 calories, 1.5 grams fat (5% of calories), 1.9 g. soluble fiber.

terol crusher. At the same time, you stock up on antioxidant vitamins C and beta-carotene, folate, flavonoids and other plant compounds. Research hints that all these may cut heart attack risk.

If you feel that this diet calls for too big a change in the way you eat, here's food for thought. Dr. Ornish says it's actually easier to stick with—because you feel so much better so quickly as a result.

Clobber Cholesterol— Deliciously

If you're looking to cut your cholesterol, give this healthy menu a try.

FOOD	TOTAL FAT (g.)	SOLUBLE FIBER (g.)
BREAKFAST		
1 cup cooked oat bran with cinnamon	3	3
1 small chopped apple with skin	0	1
1 cup nonfat milk	0	0
MORNING SNACK		
2 dried figs	0	1.5
2 vanilla wafers*	1.5	0
LUNCH		
2 cups minestrone	5.6	4.2
(¾ cup kidney beans)		
2 slices whole-wheat bread	2.4	0
½ cup carrot sticks*	0	1.1
AFTERNOON SNACK		
7 reduced-fat whole-wheat crackers*	3	0
1 orange	0	1.4

"But even if you're not ready for major changes," he says, "taking just one or two small steps is much better than doing nothing."

In fact, new research suggests substantial improvement from two amazingly easy steps. In one recent study, a group of healthy men who switched from 3 meals a day to 6 small meals or snacks averaged an 8 percent reduction in total cholesterol levels—theoretically reducing heart attack risk by

FOOD	TOTAL FAT (g.)	SOLUBLE FIBER (g.)
DINNER		
1½ cups whole-wheat spaghetti*	1.2	0
1 cup marinara sauce	1	0
1½ cups tossed mixed salad, including ½ cup shredded carrots*	0	1.1
2 tablespoons fat-free dressing*	0	0
EVENING SNACK		
Pronto Pinto Chips (see page 89)*	1.5	1.9
TOTAL	**19.2**	**15.2**

NOTE: Also contains 1,762 calories (10% of calories from fat), 5 g. saturated fat (3% of calories), 2.3 g. trans-fatty acids (1.3% of calories), 4 mg. cholesterol.

*For men, double the portion of these foods to reach 2,569 calories with 26.4 g. total fat (9% of calories), 6 g. saturated fat (2% of calories), 4.6 g. trans-fatty acids (2% of calories), 4 mg. cholesterol, 19.3 g. soluble fiber.

16 percent. Why frequent mini-meals may lower cholesterol is not yet known, but previous studies (using 9 or 17 meals a day) have shown similar drops.

And if you're still drinking whole milk, simply making the switch to skim milk could chop your cholesterol levels 7 percent, another study shows. You say you just can't drink that "blue stuff"? We'll show you how to make skim milk look and taste as creamy as 2 percent or better. (See "Stop Singin' the Skim Milk Blues".)

In fact, it's easy to topple *all* the top sources of fat in the American diet by making strategic switches at the supermarket and in the kitchen. Use four tablespoons of fat-free salad dressing instead of regular, and you save 32 grams of fat. Every tablespoon of fat-free margarine you substitute for regular saves you 10 grams of fat. That leaves you room to fill up on vegetables, fruits, grains and beans—to your heart's content!

Stop Singin' the Skim Milk Blues

Whole milk and even 2 percent "low-fat" milk have too much fat for a heart-smart diet. But if you've been shunning nonfat milk because the taste or the blue tinge has put you off, here's the perfect solution.

You can transform skim milk into a richer-tasting, creamy-looking drink with no extra fat by stirring two to four tablespoons of instant nonfat milk powder into each cup of skim until it dissolves. (The bonus is you'll be getting extra calcium! Some research links higher calcium intake with lower cholesterol levels.) In certain areas you may find skim milk in your supermarket's dairy case already fortified with nonfat milk solids—sometimes it's labeled as protein-fortified.

Constipation
How to Get Things Moving Again

DOCTORS AGREE: THE BEST MEDICINE in the world for some gastrointestinal ills is—you guessed it—diet.

So often nothing beats a strategic diet in long-term effectiveness, gentleness and convenience. This is especially true in the case of mild-to-moderate constipation. (If you suffer from more serious, persistent constipation, see your doctor.) *Prevention* magazine's healing diet for this malady consists of:

- Consuming at least 20 to 35 grams a day of dietary fiber consisting of both soluble and insoluble fiber.
- Drinking six to eight eight-ounce glasses a day of water—or the equivalent in juices, soups, skim milk and the like.
- Limiting caffeine and alcohol.

Fiber by Any Other Name . . .

It's no surprise that dietary fiber is important in relieving constipation. But what is surprising is that the type of fiber doesn't seem to matter. Formerly, soluble fiber (prevalent in legumes, oat bran, figs, mangoes, oranges and barley) was thought only to lower cholesterol without much effect on the digestive tract. Insoluble fiber (abundant in whole-wheat bran cereals) was thought to be the only type of fiber that could help out down below.

"When it comes to constipation, fiber is fiber," says William B. Ruderman, M.D., chairman in the Department of Gastroenterology at the Cleveland Clinic, Florida, in Fort Lauderdale. "It helps decrease transit time, softens the stool and adds bulk."

Says Dr. Ruderman, "I tell my patients to shoot for a total of at least 20 grams a day—though some may require less to stay regular." Twenty grams of fiber a day is the equivalent of roughly one serving of bran flakes cereal, five servings of fruits and vegetables and one serving of cooked dry lentils each day. "In reality, 20 grams a day is not always very easy to obtain day after day. It takes some planning ahead."

But add fiber slowly. Suddenly increasing fiber intake can cause uncomfortable bloating and gas. The answer is simple: "Add fiber very gradually. If you currently eat 12 grams of fiber a day, go to 15 to 17 grams each day for two weeks, then up your daily intake to 18 to 22 grams for another two weeks, and so on," says Dr. Ruderman. "Increase fiber over a period of one to three months. A lifetime of low-fiber intake can't be fixed in a week."

Spread out high-fiber foods over the whole day to avoid cramps, discomfort and possible intestinal obstruction. (High-fiber snacks such as whole-grain foods, fruits, vegetables and bran cookies can also help you meet your quota.) And if you do need to take a fiber supplement, make sure to spread those doses out, too. If you need to take two doses, take one in the morning and another at night. Lifestyle changes like diet and exercise may be easier than fiber supplements to maintain over the long haul, says Dr. Ruderman, because some people find them easier to incorporate into their daily lives.

Over-the-counter antigas drops or tablets (the product Beano is one example) taken before a meal may also help your system adjust to fiber, though hard scientific evidence remains lacking. And here's a surprise: "Some people actually have less gas when they add fiber," says Dr. Ruderman.

Lead Yourself to Water

Dehydration is a common contributor to constipation; fluids help keep things moving. "Many people simply aren't getting enough fluids," says Dr. Ruderman. "A tendency toward inadequate hydration may be endemic to our busy, caffeine-using society."

Unfortunately, thirst is a poor indicator of how much fluid you need. You may never feel thirsty and still be a little on the dry side. Yet there are lots of ways to meet the daily quota of fluids. Plain water, soups, juices, liquid dairy products, broth—all these count.

But, says Dr. Ruderman, beverages containing alcohol or caffeine cause your body to excrete fluid. If you do drink caffeine-containing or alcoholic beverages, compensate by drinking extra fluids.

This diet of fiber and fluid really works. (Regular exercise is also an important part of eliminating constipation.) "Ninety percent of people with a tendency toward mild constipation get better with the simple measures of fiber, fluid and exercise," says Dr. Ruderman.

Stewed Fruit

1 cup pitted prunes

1 cup dried apricots

1 cup raisins

Place the prunes, apricots and raisins in a pot and add just enough water to cover.

Cover and cook over low heat, simmering for 30 to 60 minutes, until the mixture is thoroughly cooked. (The ingredients will be soft.)

Remove from the heat, let cool completely, then refrigerate. Serve as a snack or dessert.

MAKES FOUR ½-CUP SERVINGS

 Nutritional Information

Per serving: 282 calories, 0.5 g. fat (2% of calories), 7.2 g. dietary fiber.

A Menu to Keep You Going

If your digestive system needs a little nudge to get going some mornings, here's a day's worth of eats to get you started.

FOOD	TOTAL FIBER (g.)
BREAKFAST	
½ oat bran bagel*	2
2 tablespoons light cream cheese*	0
1 tablespoon chopped walnuts*	0.4
1 cup Cheerios	3
½ cup 1% low-fat milk	0
½ banana, sliced	1
¾ cup orange juice*	0
1 cup decaffeinated coffee	0
LUNCH	
1¼ cups mixed spinach salad with 2 tablespoons reduced-calorie creamy Italian dressing*	4
2 tablespoons roasted sunflower seeds	1.1
1 cup lentil soup	7
¾ cup apple juice*	0
1 cup water	0
SNACK	
1 cup blueberry low-fat yogurt	1
2 vanilla wafers	0
1 cup decaffeinated herbal tea	0

FOOD	TOTAL FIBER (g.)
DINNER	
½ cup frozen broccoli spears, boiled	3
Green Giant Harvest Burger with tomato and onion	5
2 slices reduced-fat cheese	0
1 hamburger roll	1
½ cup apple sauce, unsweetened*	1
½ cup white grape juice	1
DESSERT	
1 cup decaffeinated herbal tea	0
1 peach*	1.4
1 cup low-fat frozen yogurt*†	0
TOTAL	**31.9**

NOTE: Also contains 1,796 calories with 46 g. fat (23% of calories) and over 7 cups fluid (56 ounces).

*For men, double the portion of these foods to reach 2,599 calories with 65 g. fat (23% of calories), 40.7 g. fiber and over 8½ cups fluid (68 ounces).

†For 2,600-calorie diet only.

....

Dental Health
The Top Five Toothsome Foods

YOU'RE PROBABLY WELL AWARE that some foods, particularly sweet and sticky ones, are bad for your teeth. But now here's a twist: Experts have identified foods that can actually boost your dental health—that can help *prevent* tooth decay, gum disease and other troubles. "In fact, selecting more nutritious foods is probably as important as staying away from cavity-causing foods, such as sugar and other sticky foods," says Dominick DePaola, D.D.S., Ph.D., president and dean of Baylor College of Dentistry in Dallas.

Getting proper amounts of vitamins and minerals through your diet is especially important when you're young. Nutrients play a vital role in the development of teeth, salivary glands and the surrounding structures. But even as an adult, eating nutrient-rich foods—such as fruits and vegetables, whole grains, legumes, lean meats and fish and low-fat dairy products—may help keep your mouth healthy.

Some foods do pack more of a punch than others, either because they're especially good sources of vitamins and minerals that affect your dental health or because they have special tooth decay–fighting properties. So choose the foods listed below more often, but be careful not to go overboard. Foods left too long on teeth (especially foods—such as crackers—that contain fermentable sugars) can accelerate decay. And remember: Eating more of these foods can't substitute for daily brushing and flossing and twice-a-year visits to your dentist for checkups and cleanings.

Cheese. Within the first five minutes of a sugary snack, nibble on an ounce of low-fat or nonfat cheese. That can neutralize the production of cavity-causing acids. After you eat sweets, the acidity in your mouth naturally rises, which causes tooth enamel to dissolve faster than your body can replenish it. "The net result is that you get a hole in your tooth," says Dr. DePaola. Eating a bit of aged cheese such as Cheddar or Monterey Jack stimulates the flow of saliva, which contains buffers to neutralize the acids. It's also believed that some specific components in cheese, including its calcium content, may keep enamel from dissolving.

A crisp, juicy apple. Eat raw, crunchy fruits and vegetables. "Because they contain a lot of fiber and they're crunchy, they scrape away some of the bacteria and plaque, so you get a cleansing benefit just from eating them," says Heidi K. Hausauer, D.D.S., president of the California Academy of General Dentistry and an instructor in the Department of Operative Dentistry at the University of the Pacific School of Dentistry in San Francisco.

Plus, all that chewing action exercises the gums and ligaments around the teeth, which stimulates new blood flow to the area.

Spicy foods. Try a lively salsa or toss a handful of jalapeño peppers (or as many as you can tolerate) on your next slice of low-fat pizza. You might not like the way chili peppers make your eyes water, but they make your mouth water, too, and that excess saliva helps neutralize cavity-causing acids and clean your teeth. Chilies also contain a good amount of vitamin C, a nutrient necessary for strong gums. "Vitamin C aids in the formation of collagen, which gives structure to the gum tissue and is necessary for proper healing," Dr. Hausauer says.

Plain, nonfat yogurt. It's a great source of calcium, which not only helps build strong teeth when you're young but also fortifies the bone that supports your adult pearly whites. Skip the sugary, fruited yogurts and mix plain, nonfat yogurt with fresh fruit. It's also a great baked potato topper and base for dips.

Carrots. They're full of beta-carotene. Some studies suggest that people whose diets are high in beta-carotene have a lower risk of oral cancer than people who have a lower intake of the nutrient.

In fact, in one study of people with leukoplakia—the white lesions in the mouth that can be a precursor of oral cancer—30 milligrams of beta-carotene a day produced improvement in up to 70 percent of cases, says Harinder S. Garewal, M.D., Ph.D., assistant director of cancer prevention and control, section of hematology-oncology at the Veterans Administration Hospital and the Arizona Cancer Center, both in Tucson.

Depression
Eat to Feel Better, Not Blue

AT ONE TIME OR ANOTHER, most people turn to food for solace, comfort or relaxation. One person may snack from the refrigerator at the end of a stressful day. Another might find comfort in a pint of ice cream when alone on a Friday night. Yet another may relieve her midmorning doldrums with a cinnamon roll.

In most cases the indulgence is harmless and comforting. In an effort to feel better, however, some people choose foods that unknowingly make them feel worse and set up a vicious cycle of depression and overeating. If food is making you blue, there is something you can do about it.

Might Carbohydrates Mellow Your Mood?

It is no coincidence that people want pasta, desserts and other carbohydrate-rich foods when they feel down in the dumps. Carbohydrates have a profound effect on numerous body chemicals that regulate how a person feels and acts.

Some experts have proposed that carbohydrates elevate brain levels of tryptophan and serotonin, which in turn alleviate irritability and elevate mood. A carbohydrate-rich snack of crackers and fruit, a candy bar or a whole-wheat bagel alters brain chemistry and provides temporary relief from mild depression. In contrast, a high-protein snack such as a turkey sandwich or a hamburger reduces tryptophan and serotonin levels in the brain by supplying more of the competing amino acids. Consequently, carbohydrate-sensitive people who eat a high-protein breakfast of eggs and bacon may experience mood swings and crave a doughnut by midmorning in an effort to raise brain serotonin levels and "feel better."

Interestingly, several conditions associated with depression—including premenstrual syndrome and seasonal affective disorder—are linked to increased cravings for carbohydrate-rich foods, suggesting that people unknowingly self-regulate their moods with food. Despite the supporting evidence, the carbohydrate-serotonin-depression connection remains controversial. Several studies report no differences in mood resulting from eating a high-protein or a high-carbohydrate meal. Some studies show that carbohydrates elevate serotonin levels, but fail to show any connection with mood. It may be that a certain degree of carbohydrate sensitivity is needed before symptoms are obvious enough to be measured in a scientific study. Or it could be that there is more to the food-mood connection than just serotonin.

Insidious Sugar

Research conducted by Larry Christensen, Ph.D., chairman of the Department of Psychology at the University of South Alabama in Mobile, shows that sugar and starches have different mood-altering effects even though they both stimulate serotonin production. Dr. Christensen concludes that depression often vanishes when sugar (and caffeine) are removed from the diet. "We see improvements in mood when sugar is eliminated, even in people who are not depressed; however, these sugar-sensitive people probably would have become depressed in the future," he says. Using sugar to self-regulate mood is a temporary fix. In the long run it could start a vicious cycle. "The person suffering from depression who turns to sugary foods may relieve the depression and feel better for a short while, but the depression returns," says Dr. Christensen. The person then must either reach for another sugar fix or seek help elsewhere. As opposed to the temporary sugar high, eliminating sugar and caffeine from the diet is a permanent solution to depression for some people.

Some people are so sensitive to sugar that even a small serving of something sweet, such as a cookie, sends them on a mood-swing roller coaster. These supersensitive people should eliminate all sugar from their diets, including the hidden sugars in convenience foods such as ketchup, canned fruit, fruit drinks and fruited yogurt. Other people have a higher tolerance and experience symptoms only after eating a large amount of sugar. They should cut back on concentrated sugars in candy, cakes and other desserts but might be able to tolerate the hidden sugars.

How sugar affects moods is poorly understood. One theory is that concentrated sugars in the diet raise blood glucose above normal levels, which somehow interferes with glucose transport into the cells and tissues or triggers oversecretion of insulin from the pancreas, which drops blood sugar below normal levels. Since glucose is the primary energy source for most body processes, limiting its entry essentially would starve the cells. Low blood sugar levels can also affect mood. In either case, a person feels depressed and lethargic.

A second theory is based on the connection between sugar and the endorphins—those naturally occurring morphinelike compounds in the brain responsible for euphoric feelings. If sugar does trigger a temporary release of these pleasure-producing chemicals, then turning to sweets is literally a form of unconscious self-medication. Again, however, the temporary high is usually followed by a more serious crash as blood sugar, endorphins and other hormones and chemicals drop.

Also, the more sugar you eat, the more likely your diet will be low in essential vitamins and minerals. It could be that marginal intake of one or more of these nutrients, such as magnesium or vitamin B_6, could be contributing to low energy and depression.

Don't Worry, "B" Happy

Another likely reason for a blue day is inadequate intake of one or more vitamins. Vitamin B$_6$ is a case in point. Dietary intake of this B vitamin is often marginal in many segments of the population, including women of childbearing age, children and seniors.

Confusion and depression are well-documented and common, yet vague, symptoms of vitamin B$_6$ deficiency. In one study conducted at Harvard Medical School and the Jean Mayer USDA Human Nutrition Research Center on Aging at Tufts University in Boston, more than one out of every four

Sidestepping Sweets

Most Americans consume 21 percent of their daily calories as sugar. While exact recommendations have not been set, it is generally agreed that people should cut their intake of added sugar in half—10 percent of total calories or less. So while you're cutting back on sweets such as doughnuts, cookies and ice cream, try these suggestions as well.

• Drink no more than one soft drink a day; they contain up to nine teaspoons of sugar per serving. Colas also contain caffeine.

• Read labels. While manufacturers are not required to list the percentage of sugar calories, you can get an idea of the sugar content from the ingredients list. A food may be too sweet if sugar is one of the first three ingredients or if the list includes several sources of sugar.

• Use more spices. Cinnamon, vanilla, spearmint and anise give sweet tastes to foods without adding sugar or calories. Aspartame can also be used in moderation.

depressed patients was deficient in vitamins B_6 and B_{12}. In fact, vitamin B_6 deficiency is reported in as many as 79 percent of patients with depression, compared with only 29 percent of other patients. In many cases giving these patients vitamin B_6 supplements (in doses as low as ten milligrams a day) raises vitamin B_6 levels in the blood and improves or even alleviates the depression, providing convincing evidence that the deficiency might be the cause, rather than the effect, of the depression.

Granted, overt vitamin B_6 deficiency is rare in the United States. But even a marginal intake—a person consumes enough of the vitamin to avoid classic symptoms, but not enough to sustain optimal health—could produce subtle changes in personality and mood.

Marginal intake of vitamin B_6 is compounded by medication, intense exercise, chronic dieting, alcohol consumption and/or increased nutrient needs during times of illness or stress. To increase dietary intake of the B vitamin, include several servings daily of protein-rich foods, such as chicken, nuts, legumes and fish, as well as bananas, avocados and dark green, leafy vegetables. Whole grains are preferable to refined grains, since more than 70 percent of the vitamin is lost during processing.

Always consult a physician knowledgeable about nutrition before taking vitamin B_6 supplements in doses greater than 150 milligrams for long periods of time.

More Sad-Proofing Nutrients

Vitamin B_6 is not the only deficiency that can bring you down. Marginal deficiencies of the other B vitamins, including vitamin B_1, vitamin B_2, niacin, folic acid and vitamin B_{12}, and vitamin C have been linked to depression. Large doses of vitamin A have also been implicated in some cases.

Folic acid. Folic acid deficiency is considered the most common vitamin deficiency in the United States, and intake approaching half the 1980 Recommended Dietary Allowance (RDA, now Daily Value, or DV) of 400 micrograms is probably common. A deficiency of this B vitamin—essential for normal cell growth and maintenance—causes several personality changes, including depression.

One study of healthy people between the ages of 25 and 83 showed that those with the highest blood levels of folic acid also had the best moods, while those with "low-normal" blood folic acid levels were more likely to suffer from depression. Giving these people either folic acid or a placebo improved mood in the depressed people who took the folic acid but not in the placebo group, suggesting that the depression was caused by marginal folic acid intake and was not psychosomatic. Some evidence suggests that folic acid raises serotonin levels, while a deficiency of the B vitamin results in lowered serotonin levels and increased risk of depression.

Vitamin B₁₂. People who consume marginal amounts of vitamin B_{12} are most likely to have depression and memory problems and even experience paranoia. Increased dietary or supplemental intake of B_{12} in these deficient people raises blood levels of the vitamin and appears to elevate mood.

Minerals. Low dietary intake of many of the minerals, including calcium, iron, magnesium, selenium and zinc, is reported to cause depression, irritability or mood swings.

Researchers at the University College in Swansea, Wales, assessed the moods of 50 people, then gave them either a placebo or a 100-microgram supplement of selenium. After five weeks, the selenium-supplemented people showed greater improvements in mood than did the people who took a placebo.

The degree of mood change was directly related to the person's initial selenium status; that is, the people with the lowest initial selenium intake also reported the most depression and anxiety and showed the greatest mood improvement after taking the selenium supplements.

Iron deficiency is common in active women, children and the elderly and can cause depression associated with fatigue. There is little or no evidence, however, that people already optimally nourished will benefit from additional amounts of minerals.

Are You Getting Enough B$_6$?

To determine your B$_6$ status, answer the following questions yes or no, then check your score at the end.

_____ 1. Do you eat at least 2,500 calories a day of a variety of minimally processed, wholesome foods?

_____ 2. Do you eat at least six servings daily of whole-grain breads, cereals (especially oatmeal), pasta or rice?

_____ 3. Do you frequently eat bananas, avocados, baked potatoes (including the skin), acorn squash or spinach?

_____ 4. Do you frequently eat cooked, dried beans and peas, such as lentils, lima beans, kidney beans and white beans?

_____ 5. Do you choose chicken rather than red meat, fish rather than lamb and crab rather then lunchmeats?

Give yourself two points for every yes answer and deduct two points for every no answer to the above questions. Then continue to answer either yes or no to the following questions.

_____ 6. Are you taking birth control pills, hormone replacement therapy (HRT), an anti-Parkinson's drug such as levodopa, an anti-tuberculosis drug or an anti-Wilson's drug such as D-penicillamine?

_____ 7. Do you drink more than five alcoholic beverages a week?

_____ 8. Do you eat a high-fat diet or consume several sweets and desserts daily?

Deduct one point for every yes answer and add one point for every no answer to questions 6 through 8. Then total your answers for a final score.

SCORING

10 to 13 points: Your diet is probably adequate in vitamin B_6. Consider increasing your dietary intake of vitamin B_6–rich foods or taking a supplement (with a physician's approval and monitoring) if you suspect larger-than-normal amounts of this vitamin might help alleviate PMS-related depression.

7 to 9 points: Your diet may be marginal in vitamin B_6. Add two or more of the following foods to your daily diet: bananas, avocados, chicken without skin, salmon, potato with skin, collard greens, brown rice, wheat germ, oatmeal and cornmeal. If you choose to supplement, find a multiple vitamin and mineral preparation that contains approximately two to five milligrams of vitamin B_6.

Less than 7 points: Your diet is likely to be deficient in vitamin B_6. Add three or more of the vitamin B_6–rich foods listed above to your daily diet. If you choose to supplement, follow the suggestion given above.

Fast Food Can Slow You Down

You're in a hurry and forget to pack a lunch, so once again you pull up to a drive-up window and grab a hamburger, french fries and diet soda. The meal might soothe a grumbling stomach, but it just might be why you're fighting the blues.

Granted, there is no research linking a high-fat diet with depression. This fast-food meal is a loser, however, when it comes to the vitamins and minerals that help boost spirits. For example, the meal supplies almost a third of an average woman's calorie requirement, but only 14 percent of her RDA for folic acid and less than 10 percent of her vitamin C needs. Other B vitamins also are in short supply compared with the large caloric debt.

If you are a fast-food junkie, try to gradually reduce the number of meals eaten away from home, with the long-range goal of limiting weekly fast-food meals to no more than three. Also, when you do eat at a fast-food restaurant, make better choices and supplement those choices with nutritious foods brought from home. For example, some fast-food restaurants offer lower-fat alternatives to their high-fat hamburgers that can be part of a nutritious meal if complemented with 1 percent low-fat milk, an orange and a sackful of carrots brought from home. Or you can choose salad bars or packaged green salads (with low-fat dressing) rather than a taco salad with a fried tortilla shell and too much dressing. But don't bother with the batter-fried chicken nuggets or fish: The nuggets can have as much fat as five pats of butter, while some fish fillet sandwiches have up to 29 grams of fat.

Blues-Free Basics

First, review your eating habits of the past few months. Have you been dieting, frequently skipping breakfast, eating too many sweets or eating fewer than three times a day? Any of these habits will alter your brain chemistry and possibly contribute to mood swings. Also, try to observe the following suggestions.

INDULGE YOUR CARB CRAVINGS. If you crave carbohydrates, work with—not against—your cravings.

Make sure that every meal contains some foods rich in complex carbohydrates. Breakfast can include French toast, waffles, pancakes, cereal, toast or an English muffin. Lunch and dinner can feature pasta or rice dishes, bagels and cheese. Snacks should be fruits, crackers, bread or starchy vegetables or yogurt. Also plan a carbohydrate-rich snack, such as whole-grain breads and cereals or a starchy vegetable, such as a potato or a sweet potato, for that time of the day when you are most vulnerable.

SHUN SUGAR. Replace sugary foods with nutrient-packed foods such as fruit, crunchy vegetables, whole-grain raisin bagels or low-fat yogurt.

Also, if you are fighting depression and you know you are sensitive to sugar, you should avoid all foods that contain sugar, including sugar-coated cereals, sugar-sweetened beverages and sugary snack foods such as granola bars. Read labels, since many unsuspected foods contain sugar, including muffins, canned and boxed fruit juices, frozen breakfast foods and yogurt.

CURB CAFFEINE. Try eliminating coffee, tea, cola and other caffeinated beverages, foods and medications from your diet. Bear in mind that it may take three weeks or more after you have eliminated sugar and caffeine from your diet before you notice an improvement in mood.

"EAT" YOUR VITAMINS. Keep an eye on your intake of vitamin B_6, folic acid and vitamin B_{12}.

Make sure that you include at least two folic acid–rich foods in your diet every day—that is, mix spinach with scrambled eggs for breakfast, drink at least one glass of orange juice during the day, steam collard greens and mix them into mashed potatoes or replace iceberg lettuce with folic acid–rich romaine lettuce in salads. Also, purchase vegetables fresh, refrigerate them immediately and use them within two days. Avoid overcooking dark green, leafy vegetables and always cook them in a minimum of water; then add the cooking water to soups and stews.

If Depression Doesn't Fade Away . . .

A multitude of factors can contribute to depression. Stressful events such as loss of a family member or friend, a difficult change in job or finances and problems at home or at work play a part. Medical conditions underlying depression may include changes in blood sugar, low thyroid or irregularities in blood or urine. Even a history of food sensitivities, physical problems related to foods—such as skin or respiratory problems—or a family history of allergies might contribute to the blues.

In short, what you eat is only part of the battle against the blues. Regular exercise, effective coping skills, a strong social support system and limiting or avoiding alcohol, cigarettes and medications that compound an emotional problem are important steps.

Always consult a physician if emotional problems persist or if they interfere in the long term with the quality of your life and health. In the meantime, keep in mind that what you choose to soothe your hunger will also be fueling your mood.

Diabetes
Stop Singing the Blood Sugar Blues

AFTER DECADES OF DENIAL, people with diabetes can now have their cake and wash it down with a bottle of bubbly. That's the misleading message conveyed by some headlines reporting the American Diabetes Association's (ADA) recently revised dietary guidelines. So before you start celebrating, there's a lot more that you should know about what this report says—and what it doesn't.

The overriding goal of any nutrition prescription for diabetes is to reduce complications by achieving better blood sugar control and keeping a lid on blood lipids such as cholesterol and triglycerides, says Marion Franz, R.D., director of nutrition at the International Diabetes Center in Minneapolis and co-chair of the ADA guidelines committee.

Sounds simple enough. But diet options now run the gamut from ultra low fat to 40 percent fat, with endless variations. Much depends on your particular condition, weight and lipid profile. If you don't have a good dietitian to help guide you, start looking now. You're going to need one. In the meantime, here are some basic parameters.

Can't Shake the Weight? Look at What You're Drinking

People with diabetes are often thirsty and can quaff down a steady flow of juice or soda without realizing how many calories they're taking in. "People can drink hundreds or even thousands of calories a day," says John Buse, M.D., Ph.D., assistant professor of medicine and director of the Diabetes Clinic at the University of North Carolina at Chapel Hill and former director of the endocrine clinics at the University of Chicago.

Here's the approximate calorie count on some popular beverages:

• Apple, grapefruit and orange juice—115 calories per 8 ounces
• Grape juice—150 calories per 8 ounces
• Cranberry juice cocktail—140 calories per 8 ounces
• Soda—150 calories per 12 ounces

Instead of juice, substitute water with a slice of lime or lemon, unsweetened iced tea, seltzer or soda water or just plain water, suggests Dr. Buse. If you drink sodas, choose the low-calorie varieties.

Overweight, Type I or Type II. Start with a sensible weight-loss diet, preferably lower in fat, moderate in carbohydrate intake and lower in calories. Divide daily caloric intake equally over the course of three meals and snacks.

Note: Be sure to have blood glucose and lipids monitored; increasing carb intake can sometimes elevate triglycerides or alter insulin needs.

Normal weight, high cholesterol, Type I or Type II. Start with an ultra low fat (10 percent of calories) diet that focuses on complex carbohydrates (75 percent) from grains, vegetables, beans and fruits (high in soluble fiber). Divide your daily calories over the course of three mini-meals plus three snacks.

Normal weight, high triglycerides and high VLDL (very low density lipoproteins), Type I or Type II. Consider a higher-fat diet (35 to 40 percent of calories from fat), primarily from monounsaturated fats, with moderate carbohydrate intake.

Normal weight, normal blood lipids, Type I or Type II. Eat a healthy diet with a moderate carbohydrate intake and a moderately low fat intake. The ADA recommends 30 percent of calories from fat or less; *Prevention* magazine and some health authorities now recommend a maximum of 25 percent calories from fat.

Note: All diets for people with diabetes set protein at 10 to 20 percent of total calories and total fiber at 20 to 35 grams, the same recommended for the general public.

Weighing In to Reduce Risk

The objective for people with diabetes is maintaining control of blood glucose. One of the best ways to do this, experts agree, is eating a diet that helps them attain and maintain a reasonable body weight.

"Take a look at the Pima Indians of Northern Mexico," says James J. Kenney, R.D., Ph.D., nutrition research specialist at the Pritikin Longevity Center in Santa Monica, California. Pima Indians who eat their traditional diet consisting primarily of corn, beans and desert fruit—lots of unrefined (or whole-grain) complex carbohydrates and not a lot of fat or animal protein—are not overweight and they rarely, if ever, get diabetes.

However, Pimas living today in Arizona aren't so lucky. By the age of 50, the majority of them have developed Type II diabetes, whereas before 1930, there had not been a single case, Dr. Kenney notes. Why? The Pimas have adopted the Western lifestyle, eating more sugar and fat and exercising less. As a result, they've piled on excess pounds, he says.

In fact, 80 to 90 percent of all Americans with Type II diabetes are overweight. For them a weight-control diet is absolutely the best medicine.

Generally, the greater the weight loss, the greater the improvement in blood sugar control, insulin sensitivity and blood lipids (total cholesterol, LDL, or "bad," cholesterol and

Monos to the Max

These foods all constitute one serving of a fat high in monounsaturates.

- 1 teaspoon olive oil
- 1 teaspoon canola oil
- 1 teaspoon peanut oil
- 1 teaspoon sesame oil
- 6 whole almonds
- 5 cashews
- 5 filberts
- 2 macadamia nuts
- 10 large peanuts
- 4 pecan halves
- 13 pistachio nuts
- ⅛ avocado
- 5 large olives
- 2 teaspoons peanut butter

triglycerides drop, while HDL, or "good," cholesterol increases). "But losing just ten pounds can result in a dramatic improvement in blood sugar control," adds Edward S. Horton, Sr., M.D., medical director of the Joslin Diabetes Center in Boston. In people with Type II diabetes, medication often can be reduced or eliminated.

The diet for weight loss now recommended by the ADA is a calorie-restricted one with a range of possible fat and carbohydrate ratios. But this advice is not accepted by all researchers. Dr. Kenney, for one, favors a low-fat, high-fiber, high unrefined complex carbohydrate diet—similar in composition to the traditional diet of the Pima Indians. By restricting fat, sugar and refined carbohydrates, you naturally limit calorie intake, he explains. Yet, with all the fiber in this whole-grain diet, you won't feel hungry.

"A high unrefined carbohydrate diet low in sweets and with low-calorie density is ideal," Dr. Kenney insists. "When people eat oatmeal for breakfast, bean soup for lunch, broiled haddock with a veggie-topped baked potato for dinner, perhaps some fruit for a snack, they lose weight and their blood sugar drops. If they exercise, too, their Type II diabetes almost always goes away."

What about Sweets?

That brings us to the sugar issue. Recent research has challenged the theory that sweets are metabolized faster than starches, resulting in a spike in blood sugar. It now appears that, gram for gram, the simple sugar in cakes and cookies is processed in the body in much the same way as the starch in rice, potatoes and bread. What's important, says the ADA, is the total amount of carbohydrates consumed, not the source.

In practical terms, however, substituting simple sugars for starches is anything but simple.

"An apparently small amount of concentrated sweets often contains much more carbohydrate than you think," says Christopher Saudek, M.D., director of the Johns Hopkins Diabetes Center in Baltimore.

"The point is, you don't eat a gram of concentrated sweets like you would a gram of complex carbohydrate," he explains. "That's the big danger, and that's why I urge people with diabetes to avoid concentrated sweets." Each time you choose a sweet over a starchy grain or vegetable, you sacrifice nutrition and satiety. Three tablespoons of honey equals a whole potato in grams of carbohydrate, for example.

Another stumbling block: It's next to impossible to know how many carbohydrates are in homemade baked goods and treats from the corner bakery. There are no labels or recommended serving sizes to guide you.

(continued on page 118)

Dial "D" for Dietitian

If you have diabetes, what you eat—and don't eat—can have a profound effect on your health and well-being. That's why some doctors recommend having a dietitian in your corner, too.

"The old idea of a doctor or a doctor's secretary handing a person with diabetes a preprinted diet sheet is out," says Christopher D. Saudek, M.D., director of the Johns Hopkins Diabetes Center in Baltimore. Instead, doctors recommend that people with diabetes work with a dietitian. "This is particularly critical for someone with Type I (insulin-dependent) diabetes," says Dr. Saudek, "because changes in diet may have a profound effect on insulin requirements and should be done with caution."

The dietitian will review medical needs, diet history and eating habits as well as lifestyle, work habits and culture before devising an individualized meal plan. As always, people with diabetes should regularly monitor their blood glucose and lipid levels with their physicians.

A Mono-Rich Meal Plan

Adding more monounsaturated fats to your diet is simpler—and tastier—than you might think. Take a look at the sample menu below designed by Joyce P. Barnett, R.D., a dietitian at the University of Texas Southwestern Medical Center at Dallas.

FOOD	MONO-UNSATURATED FAT (g.)
BREAKFAST	
I cup 1% low-fat milk	0.75
¾ cup wheat flakes	0
½ banana	0
I slice whole-wheat toast	0.35
I tablespoon peanut butter	3.78
I bran muffin prepared with canola oil*	4.17
LUNCH	
I cup 1% low-fat milk	0.75
4 ounces cooked lean beef	2.25
I cup stir-fried broccoli with I tablespoon peanut oil	6.28
15 cashews	6.95
⅔ cup steamed white rice	0
I orange	0
SNACK	
12 almonds*	7
DINNER	
3 ounces chicken breast sautéed in 2 teaspoons olive oil	7.69
plus I ounce chicken*	1.05

FOOD	MONO-UNSATURATED FAT (g.)
½ cup mashed potatoes	1.86
1 teaspoon margarine	1.49
½ cup green beans	0
½ cup cauliflower*	0
Salad of 1 cup raw zucchini marinated with 2 teaspoons olive oil, and 5 large olives	8.38
1 slice whole-wheat bread*	0.35

SNACK

1 small apple	0
¼ cup 2% low-fat cottage cheese	0.31
1 slice whole-wheat bread*	0.35
1 ounce roast turkey*	0.48
1 teaspoon mayonnaise*	0.44
4 pecan halves*	3.4
TOTAL	**40.84**

NOTE: Contains 1,826 calories with 77 g. total fat (38% of calories) and 20% of calories from monounsaturated fat.

*For men, add these foods to increase calories to 2,623 with 112 g. total fat (39% of calories) and 58.08 g. monounsaturated fat (20% of calories).

Finally, don't lose sight of the fact that sweets in combination with fats are caloric heavyweights. And weight management is a primary treatment for many—if not most—people with diabetes. The bottom line? Yes, you may be able to include sweets as part of a carefully planned diabetes diet. But the truth is, it's a lot easier to maintain blood sugar control without them. At most, treat sweets as very occasional treats, not everyday foods. The same goes for alcohol. Although the ADA guidelines allow that people with well-controlled diabetes can indulge in a drink or two with meals, not everyone with diabetes can or should, cautions John Buse, M.D., Ph.D., assistant professor of medicine and director of the Diabetes Clinic at the University of North Carolina at Chapel Hill and former director of the endocrine clinics at the University of Chicago.

Alcohol is a carbohydrate that is metabolized in the body as a fat. So a bottle of beer or a glass of wine counts as two fat exchanges (ten grams of fat, or 90 calories). As a calorie-laden, nutritionally lacking food, alcohol is a poor choice for any person with or without diabetes who's watching his weight. If you have high triglycerides or low blood sugar problems, extra caution is advised. Alcohol can drive up triglycerides, and if consumed without food, it can cause a drop in blood sugar levels.

High Triglycerides? Talk to Your Doctor

If your diabetes is complicated by high fasting triglycerides (greater than 250), the newest ADA guidelines suggest that you might want to take a different nutrition approach. Because high-carbohydrate diets have a tendency to elevate triglycerides in some people, this may be a situation in which higher fat is the way to go, says Dr. Horton. You should not, however, follow this diet unless your doctor advises you to.

These guidelines suggest that, if this is your situation, you may want to try a 40 percent fat-calorie diet; half the fat should be monounsaturated. A dietitian can help you with food selections for this diet. (See the sample monounsaturated-fat diet on page 116.)

A study in Denmark found that blood pressure fell and

blood sugar control improved in patients who ate a diet that was 50 percent fat with 30 percent of those calories coming from monounsaturated fats. Other studies have indicated that a diet high in monounsaturated fats brought down triglyceride levels.

There's just one thing to watch with a diet like this: your weight. Make sure that when you increase calories from fat, you don't increase total calories.

....

Fatigue
Get Back That Get-Up-and-Go

YOUR DAYS FEEL LIKE a dawn-to-dusk dance marathon: Up with the sun, you marshal the troops out the door and grab a quick doughnut and coffee to munch in the car. With a full day of work ahead, a quick burger is all you can manage for lunch. A battle with the 3 o'clock slump, and suddenly it's time to race home, cook dinner and survive an evening of laundry, kids' homework, the Cub Scouts carpool and a batch of bills to pay.

Small wonder you're feeling irritable, frustrated and decidedly unamorous—as if your brain is grinding along in low gear. You're tired. Your diet may be the reason. And if so, you're not alone.

"On any given day, one-quarter of the population is tired, and an estimated 2 to 3 percent of the entire U.S. population feels fatigue that's nearly disabling," says Richard Podell, M.D., clinical professor of Family Medicine at the Robert Wood Johnson Medical School of the University of Medicine and Dentistry of New Jersey in New Brunswick and author of *Doctor, Why Am I So Tired?*. "Of these people, more are women than men. And dietary changes help about one in four feel better."

Lifestyles of the Run-Down and Fatigued

Why is fatigue one of the top ten complaints that women report to doctors? Blame it on lifestyle: Women who juggle jobs, families and households often get little sleep and less exercise. Instead of eating nutrition-packed, energy-boosting meals, we graze at salad bars and fast-food drive-throughs, missing out on essential vitamins and minerals—notably iron, B vitamins, magnesium and folic acid—needed to maintain energy.

Many women intentionally undereat in an attempt to lose weight, and they undernourish themselves in the process. Others feel drained of energy because of pregnancy, childbirth and menopause.

Some of us overeat and feel sluggish because our bodies are busy digesting and storing excess fat. That actually slows blood circulation, reducing the delivery of oxygen to the body's cells, says researcher R. James Barnard, Ph.D., professor of physiological science at the University of California, Los Angeles, and consultant to the Pritikin Longevity Center in Santa Monica, California. Or we choose the wrong foods at the wrong time—say, a bacon cheeseburger or pizza at a business lunch, or for some women, drinking large amounts of coffee instead of eating, or eating a high-fat snack such as a chocolate croissant or french fries—and feel sluggish instead of energized.

By the way, smoking, drinking and recreational drugs can also tire you out, as will a variety of conditions from anemia to diabetes to depression. If you're suddenly bone-tired for no obvious reason, or have been barely able to function for a month or longer, it's time to see a doctor.

Otherwise, you may simply need an oomph-restoring meal makeover.

Perk Up with Protein, Calm Down with Carbs

Firsthand experience has taught many women what research now reveals about food's power to boost—or flatten—energy levels.

"If I eat a big lunch," says Lydia W., "I'm mentally sluggish all afternoon. A couple of light meals during the day works better."

"There have been times when I feel tired and realize I have not been eating well," says a 32-year-old computer programmer.

If mustering mental energy—to finish a report for an afternoon deadline or work late on your income tax—is your goal, did you know that eating small amounts of protein as part of a low-fat meal plan can actually help your brain manufacture more of the neurotransmitters that make you mentally alert?

By topping your morning toast with non-fat or low-fat ricotta cheese, choosing a turkey sandwich for lunch or broiled fish for dinner, you can subtly override your natural body rhythms, fighting the built-in tendency to grow mentally tired as the day wanes and increasing your brain's high-energy time by up to three hours.

"When your mother said 'Eat fish; it's a brain food,' she wasn't that far off," says Judith Wurtman, Ph.D., nutrition research scientist at the Massachusetts Institute of Technology in Cambridge and author of *Managing Your Mind and Mood Through Food*.

It's true that we need complex carbohydrates such as pasta and whole-wheat bread to fuel muscles. But according to Dr. Wurtman's research, carbohydrates eaten alone make more of the amino acid tryptophan available to your brain. Your brain uses the tryptophan to manufacture serotonin, a nerve-transmitting substance that leaves you feeling "less stressed, less anxious and more relaxed," she says.

In contrast, protein gives your brain cells more of the amino acid tyrosine, which is converted to dopamine and norepinephrine—the very chemicals that leap from nerve ending to nerve ending inside your brain when you're engaged in thought. "Sharp thinking skills, word retrieval and mental quickness depend on protein," Dr. Wurtman says. "If you don't eat much protein, you will probably find that you're not as mentally alert."

The advice doesn't hold for everyone, Dr. Wurtman notes. A few of us are carbohydrate cravers; we may experience fatigue along with depression or tension, anger or anxiety. "For these people," she says, "eating carbohydrates does make them feel better and more focused."

Sports Drinks and Energy Bars: Real Food Will Do

Lime green, lemon yellow or dazzling orange. Sports drinks, with their high-performance promises and neon-bright fruit flavors, are popping up everywhere these days—at the gym, in the supermarket and on TV commercials. So are foil-wrapped sports energy bars. You can't miss them. But do you need them?

Probably not for most people who just work out for less than 90 minutes, says Edward Coyle, Ph.D., an exercise physiologist in the Department of Kinesiology at the University of Texas at Austin. Aerobics adherents, fitness walkers and joggers and others who work out to lose weight and stay fit can easily meet their energy and fluid needs with water and healthy snacks.

Drinks such as Gatorade, All Sport and Powerade *do* work, notes Dr. Coyle. Some sports drinks contain scientifically engineered blends of carbohydrates, sodium and—of course—water, formulated to quickly replace fluids, minerals and calories lost during sweaty exercise. "But it's nothing magic," he says. The same ingredients are found in regular food.

"There's no evidence that a moderately active woman who is exercising for one hour or less a day at below 85 percent of maximum heart rate needs the extra carbohydrates or minerals for energy or rehydration," says Dr. Coyle, who has researched sports

Food for Thought

Carbohydrates are also the body's basic brain fuel and are vital for sustaining body functions. While you can get carbohydrates in everything from beans and rice to fruits and veg-

drinks extensively. "Unless she's an endurance athlete running hard for longer than one hour or playing back-to-back sets of tennis on a really hot day, all she needs is plenty of water plus a snack or a meal within a few hours after exercising."

To stay hydrated: An hour or so before your workout, down 16 ounces of water. During your exercise routine drink another 8 ounces every 20 minutes. Afterward, weigh yourself and drink enough water to replace the weight that you've lost, says Michael Sawka, Ph.D., environmental physiologist in the Thermal Physiology and Medicine Division of the U.S. Army Research Institute of Environmental Medicine in Natick, Massachusetts.

And here's why. "You could easily lose a quart of water in an hour of exercise," Dr. Sawka says. "That's two pounds. Even that small loss can raise your body temperature and heart rate, which will make it harder for you to perform well."

As for sports bars, you can get the same 200-calorie burst of energy with "four Fig Newtons or a large banana or other similar snack," notes Nancy Clark, R.D., director of nutrition services at SportsMedicine Brookline in the Boston area. (And they're less expensive.)

etables to candy bars and soft drinks, don't be tempted by a quick sugar hit—all carbohydrates are not created equal.

"Some carbohydrates, like sugar, honey, candies and baked desserts, give you a very quick fix, but you end up being hungry and tired and back in the refrigerator eating in a matter of hours," says Elizabeth Somer, R.D., dietitian and author of *Nutrition for Women* and *Food and Mood.*

In contrast, complex carbohydrates that are also high in fiber—such as beans, vegetables and whole-grain products— may provide a steadier source of fuel for your body, says David Jenkins, M.D., Ph.D., professor of medicine and nutritional sciences at the University of Toronto.

Why? Your body digests more slowly. Meals and snacks that combine carbohydrates with small amounts of fat or protein may also provide an even release of energy for the same reason.

For snacks that combine carbohydrates, low-fat protein and fiber, try a piece of fruit with crackers and peanut butter, rice cakes with low-fat cheese or yogurt, a baked potato topped with nonfat cottage cheese, a three-bean salad or an English muffin spread with all-fruit jam and nonfat cheese, suggests Somer.

Just as important, Somer notes, is giving your body a steady fuel source that begins promptly with the first meal of the day. "You are literally breaking a fast—your body hasn't had food for the past 8 or 10 or 12 hours. If you skip breakfast you might never rebuild your energy stores for the day," she says.

Your best bet for steady energy may be smaller, more frequent meals—perhaps five a day, says Dr. Podell. "Eating a large amount of food, say, more than 1,000 calories at a meal, will typically make many people tired within 30 to 60 minutes. This is caused by neurochemical changes in the brain relating to the amino acid tryptophan. In addition, some people will experience a 'hypoglycemic' rebound three to four hours later that could make them tired and irritable. These are two distinct reactions. Some people get one or the other, and some get both reactions," he says.

Micronutrients for Macro-energy

By nature, women have special vitamin and mineral needs. Menstruation and childbirth can drain iron stores, leaving you fatigued and even anemic. So can diets bereft of rich and reliable sources of iron such as lean meats and iron-rich beans, dried fruit, shellfish and nuts.

Birth control pills can bring on deficiencies of vitamin B$_6$ and folic acid, causing a run-down feeling. Women who are on the Pill should be sure to get plenty of foods rich in vitamin B$_6$, such as wheat germ, bananas, avocados, cabbage and cauliflower and foods rich in folate, such as apricots, pumpkins, carrots, beans and green leafy vegetables like spinach to boost energy, according to Dr. Podell.

Taking diuretics and drinking too much alcohol can drain both potassium and magnesium, leaving you fatigued, with weak muscles and poor concentration. To correct it, turn to potassium-packed dried fruits, citrus, banana, green leafy vegetables and magnesium-rich nuts, seeds and green veggies, Dr. Podell suggests. And if you do take diuretics, ask your doctor about blood-potassium tests as well as diuretics that don't drain this vital nutrient.

And don't forget six to eight glasses (eight-ounce) of water a day, suggests Somer. "Fatigue is a sign of mild dehydration," she says. "We tend to go for coffee or tea to feel peppier, but the caffeine acts as a diuretic and takes water out of our bodies. Most women aren't getting enough water."

Sluggish? Ditch the Doughnuts

Speaking of caffeine, coffee and a sweet treat—a doughnut or slice of cake, for instance—may be old standbys for anyone needing a pick-me-up, but nutritionists and researchers warn that this duo just might slam-dunk your energy levels, leaving you with less vim than before.

Coffee, experts say, is a two-edged sword: research shows that caffeine improves alertness. But sipping too much—or enjoying your java too late in the day—could leave you tossing and turning on your pillow at night. And for some, even a morning cup can lead to tiredness, depression or a mid-morning slump.

"A cup of coffee in the morning will get you going and sharpen your thinking," explains Somer, who calls java the number one mind-altering drug. "But drinking more than three five-ounce cups a day, and especially drinking coffee after midday, can interfere with sleep." And as you can probably guess, poor sleep translates into below-par energy levels.

Skip the caffeine, and you may recoup your zest. In a series of studies at Texas A&M University in College Station, Larry Christensen, Ph.D., now chairman of the Department of Psychology at the University of South Alabama in Mobile, found that depressed men and women who eliminated sugar and caffeine from their diets felt more energetic and less depressed.

"If you're depressed or have constant feelings of fatigue, then it's worth trying," says Dr. Christensen. "Though I should warn you," he adds, "people went through some withdrawal giving up both sugar and caffeine. They can be hard habits to break."

In a Yale University study eight volunteers who sipped caffeine-containing sodas—the equivalent of two to three cups of drip-brewed coffee—felt dizzy and trembling and developed other typical symptoms of hypoglycemia when their blood sugar was lowered to levels that are close to hypoglycemia but do not usually produce any symptoms.

Why? Researcher Pierre Fayad, M.D., assistant professor of neurology at the Yale University School of Medicine and co-director of the Yale Vascular Neurology Program, says that the caffeine actually slowed blood flow to the brain, probably lowering the availability of sugar for the brain to use. Drinking less coffee, switching to decaf or eating food or pastries along with the coffee may help prevent a low blood sugar, says Dr. Fayad.

Want to quit entirely? Don't go cold turkey. Pour yourself one-fourth less coffee than usual per cup and continue to cut down until you've weaned yourself entirely, suggests Wahida

Karmally, R.D., director of nutrition at the Irving Center for Clinical Research at Columbia University in New York.

Or switch gradually to decaffeinated coffee. Start out by mixing three-quarters of a cup of regular brew with one-quarter decaf. Every two or three days replace a little more caffeinated with decaf until your cup's full of 100 percent decaf. "Go slowly," says Karmally, "weaning yourself off caffeine at your own pace."

Heart Disease Prevention
A Matter of Fat

İT HAPPENS 171 TIMES every hour of every day—the frantic call to 911, the desperate struggle in the ambulance or emergency room, the tears and fears and prayers for a loved one hit by heart attack. But no matter who the victim is, there's always the shocking disbelief that it "suddenly" and "unexpectedly" happened.

Actually, heart attack doesn't "just happen." Usually, it's been years in the making.

"When you compare all the factors that contribute to a heart attack, it seems as though diet is probably the most significant," says Basil Rifkind, M.D., chief of the Lipid Metabolism and Atherogenesis Branch of the National Heart, Lung and Blood Institute in Bethesda, Maryland.

"You look at countries like Japan where people smoke a great deal, have high blood pressure and live with a lot of stress. But they still have a negligible rate of coronary disease because they have much lower blood cholesterol levels," Dr. Rifkind notes. "Once your cholesterol level is high—which results from a diet high in saturated fats and cholesterol—these other factors aggravate the situation and put you at additional risk for heart disease."

You Can Cut Your Risk

Your chances of having or dying from a heart attack are greater if you are male, are over age 65 or have a family history of heart disease. Other factors that increase your risk include smoking, stress, being overweight or having diabetes, high blood pressure or high cholesterol.

A poor diet just adds to some of these risk factors—particularly when that diet contributes to obesity, high blood pressure and high cholesterol. But while the way you eat can be a cause of heart attack, researchers are learning that it can also be the cure.

"There have been major studies showing that you can reverse plaque in the arteries, and part of the therapy has been a diet low in saturated fats," says Neil Stone, M.D., associate professor of medicine at Northwestern University Medical School in Chicago and chairman of the American Heart Association (AHA) Nutrition Committee.

In fact, Dr. Stone notes that in some cases, diet alone may be as effective in reducing heart attack risk as both going on a low-fat diet and taking cholesterol-lowering medication. "At least one study showed that diet alone could produce a risk regression rate that was similar to what was accomplished previously with diet and medication."

Sleuthing Out Sneaky Fats

So the answer to reversing the risk of heart attack seems obvious enough: Follow the AHA's guidelines of getting no more than 30 percent of your overall calories from fat sources. And within those guidelines, you need to pay particular attention to which kind of fat you're getting. In order to reduce the risk of heart attack significantly, no more than 10 percent of your calories should come from saturated fats. Unfortunately, what isn't so obvious is just where all those fat calories come from.

For instance, we're told that saturated fats are associated with the clogging of arteries and can cause heart attack, and these are mostly so-called animal fats. And we're told that vegetable fats, such as monounsaturated fats, can be heart-healthy.

But what we're not always told is that some vegetable fats can do even more damage than animal fats—and many of those fats are no further away than your own kitchen shelves.

The Great Trans Wreck

Trans-fatty acids are the result of a commercial process called hydrogenation, in which cheaper (and usually heart-healthy) vegetable oils are turned into a semisolid state resembling butter. Hundreds of food manufacturers use hydrogenated ingredients to give their foods longer shelf life, more texture and a richer, more appealing taste. Foods that are most likely to contain trans-fatty acids include fast foods, baked goods, snack foods, sweets and even pizza. But what's good for the palate is nasty for the heart.

"In one study we found a twofold increase in risk of heart attack between people who had the most trans-fatty acids in their diets and those who had the least," says Alberto Ascherio, M.D., Dr.P.H., assistant professor of nutrition and epidemiology at Harvard University School of Public Health. "And other studies have had similar findings."

Some studies indicate that trans-fatty acids may do their dirty work by raising harmful low-density lipoproteins (LDLs) while possibly lowering helpful high-density lipoproteins (HDLs). And apparently, trans-fatty acids are worse than saturated fats in changing the ratio between overall cholesterol and HDL cholesterol. In fact, "they seem to increase the ratio between overall cholesterol levels and HDL cholesterol at twice the rate of saturated fats," says Lisa Litin, R.D., a research dietitian at Harvard. The more trans-fatty acids you have in your diet, the more your heart disease risk goes up. But it's not that difficult to shave a number of grams off that daily total—as long as you know where the trans-fats come from. Here's how to tell.

READ THOSE FOOD LABELS. "If you see the words *hydrogenated* or *partially hydrogenated vegetable oil,* the food contains trans-fatty acids and consumption should be limited," says Dr. Ascherio.

Another clue: "Any label that says 'May contain one or more of the following' and lists partially hydrogenated cotton-seed, soybean or other oils indicates that it's been chemically changed and contains trans-fatty acids," adds Litin.

Keep a Good Beat with Cardio-Nutrients

The right diet may be one of your best hedges against heart attack. But you should also learn to love foods that are high in certain vitamins and minerals that have been found to protect against heart disease. Among the most important:

Beta-carotene. Along with fellow antioxidant vitamins C and E, beta-carotene protects against heart attack by keeping the harmful form of cholesterol from attaching to artery walls, where it can harden and cause atherosclerosis. The benefits of beta-carotene were discovered in the Physicians Health Study at Harvard Medical School. Results from the research suggested that people who ate the most beta-carotene were only one-fourth as likely to have a heart attack as those who ate the least. Good sources of beta-carotene include sweet potatoes, mangoes, apricots, yellow squash, spinach and broccoli.

Vitamin C. Besides keeping plaque from hardening (or "oxidizing"), vitamin C has other benefits. "It can lower the levels of LDL (low-density lipoprotein, or bad, cholesterol) while increasing HDL (high-density lipoprotein, or good, cholesterol)," says Aleksandra Niedzwiecki, Ph.D., head of cardiovascular research at the Linus Pauling Institute of Science and Medicine in Palo Alto, California. "Vitamin C also helps keep artery walls healthy—and increased intake of

Remember, food labels list ingredients from highest quantity to lowest. So if you see any of these ingredients among the top three or four on the list, you know that the food product is very high in trans-fatty acids. If the hydrogenated fats are lower on the list, then the amount of trans-fatty acids in the product is probably minimal.

---

this vitamin can prevent hardening of the arteries." Some of the best sources are orange juice, cantaloupe, broccoli, brussels sprouts, green peppers, strawberries and kiwifruit.

Vitamin E. Of the three antioxidant vitamins, the big E has the best antioxidizing effect. In fact, Harvard researchers say that by taking 100 international units daily, women could cut their risk of heart disease by nearly half and men could reduce it by one-third. The only problem is that vitamin E is highest in food sources that should be used sparingly, such as cooking oils and margarine. A supplement may be your best route to get the E you need, but also try to eat pumpkin seeds, cashews, Brazil nuts, almonds, sunflower seeds and ready-to-eat cereals.

Magnesium. A high-magnesium diet after a heart attack can slash the postepisode death rate by 55 percent, report the National Institutes of Health. It may also be a good preventive, adds Forrest Nielsen, Ph.D., director of the U.S. Department of Agriculture Human Nutrition Research Center in Grand Forks, North Dakota. "A lack of dietary magnesium can lead to irregular heartbeats, and magnesium also may keep cholesterol from oxidizing, much like the antioxidant vitamins," he says. Some of the best food sources include bananas, prunes, apricots and pears.

SIDESTEP SHORTENING. "A product that boasts 100 percent vegetable shortening may sound healthy, but it's very high in trans-fatty acids," says Litin.

CHOOSE TUB MARGARINE RATHER THAN STICK. Go soft. Soft margarine has about one-third the trans-fatty acids of stick margarine.

ESCHEW FRIED FOOD. Not long ago many fast-food restaurants switched from frying foods in saturated fats such as beef tallow and tropical oils to using "healthier" 100 percent vegetable shortening. Naturally, most people assumed that their french fries and other deep-fried delights were much more heart-healthy than before. "However," says Litin, "these commercial food products contain 25 to 30 percent trans-fatty acids." Says Bruce Holub, Ph.D., a researcher and nutritionist at the University of Guelph in Ontario, Canada, "Fried foods in general, and particularly those served in fast-food restaurants, have the most trans-fats of just about any food." And, he adds, it doesn't matter which fried food you choose—fries, chicken or fish.

AVOID PREPACKAGED FOODS. Foods such as pancake mixes, ready-to-eat waffles, cookies and cakes all contain trans-fats in varying amounts, adds Dr. Holub. You can usually reduce the amount of trans-fats (and saturated fats) by making these foods yourself. "Just adapt the recipes somewhat and use cooking oils in place of margarine or butter—or use half margarine and half oil," suggests Litin.

Oil Mixed Up

Actually, cooking oils may present their own problem. Sure, some cooking oils are among the best food sources of polyunsaturated and monounsaturated fats, which can actually help reduce your risk of heart attack by lowering cholesterol. The problem is, oils are probably the single biggest source of "hidden" fats in the American diet.

"Many people think they can eat anything they want as long as they add some unsaturated salad oil. But that's not the way it is," says nutrition expert Robert Nicolosi, Ph.D., professor of clinical science and director of cardiovascular research at the University of Massachusetts in Lowell. "You have to have these oils rich in monounsaturated and polyunsaturated fats as a *substitute* for saturated fats. Unfortunately, what a lot of people do is overdo it by adding more mono- or polyunsaturated oils, thinking they're doing themselves a favor."

Don't Hold the Onion

Are you an onion-lover? Then you're in luck. The same sulfur compounds in onions that make your eyes water help raise the "good" high-density lipoprotein, or HDL, cholesterol that helps clean artery walls, says Isabella Lipinska, Ph.D., nutritional counselor for the Cardiac Rehabilitation Program at Saint Elizabeth's Hospital in Boston.

Onions also help decrease triglycerides and may also have a thinning effect on the blood that lessens the risk of blood clots. But what's most exciting about onions is that they may actually make fatty meals less dangerous.

"After you have a fatty meal there is an influx of fat entering your bloodstream, which can raise your risk of heart attack," says Dr. Lipinska. "Onions help prevent this influx of fat because of the sulfur compounds, so if you have onions with that fatty meal, you'll lessen its negative effects."

It doesn't take much—only about one medium onion a day—to get these heart-helping benefits. And to make onions even more healthy, you can "sweat" them so they can cook fat-free without butter. Just slice the onions into thick layers and lay them flat in a no-stick frying pan over medium heat. Place a lid or parchment paper on top of the slices and cover them tightly for two minutes. When the onions have beads of "sweat," they're ready to eat.

All cooking oils pack a lot of calories in a little bit—120 per tablespoon. And we tend to go overboard with cooking oil. Some people use several tablespoons of oil to coat a 12-inch frying pan when one to two teaspoons will do.

For the same reason you'd avoid these oils on a weight-loss program, you also need to avoid them for the sake of your heart. Here's how to convert your oil consumption, no matter how healthy your choice of oil.

- Stir-fry with orange juice, suggests Dr. Nicolosi. "The key, however, is to use as little oil as possible—ideally, no more than one tablespoon of oil, and preferably, just a few drops," he says. "You replace the rest with orange juice, which works very well and adds a great flavor to whatever you're cooking."
- Instead of pouring cooking oil into a pan, apply about one teaspoon with a small pastry brush or rub it on with a paper towel. This method prevents food from sticking, but you'll use a lot less oil. That alone can cut several hundred calories from a meal.
- In recipes that specifically call for very flavorful (and saturated) fats, try using no more than one-quarter of the suggested amount and make up the difference with one-quarter unsaturated vegetable oil. Then mix that oil duo half-and-half with water, vinegar or stock.
- Don't assume that "light" oil has fewer calories. The calorie content is the same in light olive oil as in other oils. *Light* refers to a milder flavor, which results from the way the oil is processed.

Why Light Products Can Pork You Out

Oils aren't the only reputed heart-healthy foods that have hidden fat. In fact, our diets are full of sneaky fat contributors, which probably explains why, in this era of lean eating, we're consuming more calories than ever before.

Despite their claims of being cholesterol-free and low in saturated fat, many items are loaded with unsuspected trans-fatty acids that increase the "bad" (LDL) cholesterol, lower the "good" (HDL) cholesterol and increase the risk of heart attack. These foods are often high in total fat, which contributes to obesity and heart disease. Here's how to avoid some of the worst offenders since the charge of the light brigade.

RECONSIDER THAT MORNING MUFFIN. Most ready-made muffins sold at supermarkets and coffee shops often have more fat than a similar-size doughnut because they're loaded with cooking oils. In addition, a store-bought muffin may be merely masquerading as healthful, since many are high in trans-fatty acids, adds Dr. Holub.

Here's one way to tell if your muffin is high in fat. Leave the muffin on a paper napkin for about ten minutes. If there's a spot on the napkin, rub it to find out if it's greasy. A grease spot means that your muffin is full of fat, so you might want to avoid that brand in the future.

AVOID FROZEN FOODS. Processed foods, TV dinners and other frozen foods tend to be very high in fat—even if they claim to be otherwise, according to nutritionists. Some frozen dinners have twice as much fat as the same dish that you'd prepare yourself. Most are also very high in sodium.

For example, a six-ounce serving of frozen pasta primavera has 305 calories and over 14 grams of fat, and it gets nearly half its calories from fat. It also has 1,410 milligrams of sodium—the entire daily requirement for some people. Make it yourself, though, using the same pasta and vegetables (but fewer of the other fatty and salty ingredients), and a six-ounce portion has only 267 calories, 7 grams of fat and 220 milligrams of sodium.

DON'T CHICKEN OUT AT FAST-FOOD JOINTS. If you're looking for a lower-fat alternative to a typical fast-food meal of a burger, fries and a milkshake, don't assume that chicken is automatically a better choice. Any fast-food chicken that's dipped in batter and fried is loaded with fat. But if you order a grilled chicken sandwich, you get less fat and fewer calories.

BELLY UP TO THE SALAD BAR. But be sure to scoop up the leafy green vegetables, cucumbers, tomatoes, carrots and broccoli. And avoid toppings such as cheese, ham, full-fat dressing and creamy goodies such as macaroni salad or potato salad. Otherwise, you're getting even more fat than you'd get in a burger. If you make the mistake of ordering a fully loaded taco salad in the shell, you're looking at 60 grams of total fat—what you'd get in four cheeseburgers!

Eat as the Romans (and French) Do

Of course, the way you eat also makes a difference. And if you don't believe it, just look at the other side of the Atlantic. The French, for instance, practically live on cheese, butter and other foods rich in saturated fats, but France still has a very low rate of heart disease.

Medical researchers call this the French Paradox. It's been puzzled over since the 1950s, when researchers first noticed that countries whose populations had the most fat in their diets tended to have the highest rates of heart disease—and then noticed that France was a glaring exception.

Several explanations were offered. First, the French traditionally drink a lot of wine, which some experts say helps raise artery-scouring HDL cholesterol. Second, the French tend to consume more vegetables and less meat. But still, the average Parisian eats more fat and cholesterol than the average Philadelphian does—yet we Americans have twice the rate of heart attack. And many other European countries have the same low rate of death from cardiovascular heart disease as France.

Researchers then considered the *way* they eat. "It's not just the American diet that's bad, but also our eating habits," says Dr. Nicolosi. "Besides reducing the saturated fats and dietary cholesterol in your diet, the way to lower the risk of heart attack, I believe, is to exercise more and practice eating habits more like Europeans'." Here's how.

DON'T WATCH THE CLOCK. "Our first mistake," says Dr. Nicolosi, "is that we eat on cue. When the clock says it's 8:00 or 9:00 A.M., we have to have breakfast. When it strikes noon, we have to have lunch. We may be eating those meals more out of habit than hunger. When you do that, you tend to eat more throughout the day than you should."

Fish for Good Health

Omega-3 fatty acids, found in many types of freshwater and saltwater fish, help lower your liver's production of VLDL (very low density lipoprotein), a particularly bad type of blood fat. Omega-3's also raise HDL (high-density lipoprotein), the good cholesterol that's been linked to protecting against heart attacks and heart disease. In addition, these fatty acids seem to reduce the tendency of blood to form clots—a leading cause of heart attack. And these fish oils have been found to prevent reblockage of arteries that have been opened by balloon angioplasty.

SEAFOOD (3 oz.)	OMEGA-3'S (g.)
Anchovies, canned in olive oil	1.8
Atlantic herring	1.8
Pink salmon, canned	1.5
Atlantic sardines, canned	1.3
Bluefin tuna	1.3
Atlantic mackerel	1.1
Sockeye salmon	1.1
Bluefish	0.8
Rainbow trout	0.8
Swordfish	0.8
Albacore tuna, canned in water	0.7
Sea bass	0.7
Freshwater bass	0.7
Pompano	0.6
Halibut	0.5
Chinook salmon (lox), smoked	0.4
Pollack	0.4
Flounder	0.2

EAT MORE, EARLY. "In the United States, a typical dinner can be at least 1,500 calories—that's way too much for late in the day," says Dr. Nicolosi. "Compare that with France and other countries, where most of the day's calories are consumed at breakfast and lunch. That gives them plenty of time to burn off their calories." By having your bigger meals early in the day, you're more likely to lose weight. Eating a lot just a few hours before sleep is a sure way to contribute to obesity.

EAT SMALLER PORTIONS. While some Europeans have plenty of fat-filled foods, many—like the French, Italians and Spaniards—just plain eat less. "They eat smaller meals than we do, which is why they don't have the obesity problem—and rate of heart attack," says Dr. Nicolosi. "In America, the most successful restaurants are those that force you to leave with a doggie bag. In Europe, the portions are smaller—probably half the size of ours."

SWITCH TO FRUIT OR LOW-FAT YOGURT FOR DESSERT. Mediterraneans usually end their meals with fresh fruit. They evade the truckloads of fat and refined sugar and get lots of vitamin C, beta-carotene and fiber.

Easy Changes, Extraordinary Results

Here are some other heart-smart strategies that help you reduce heart attack risk.

TRIM FAT. Remove the skin of chicken or turkey before you eat it. You'll avoid 71 percent of its fat content. It's fine to cook the bird with the skin on since the fat doesn't "seep" into the meat, but going skinless can slash 50 grams of fat off a typical four-pound chicken.

DON'T DEPEND ON DECAF. Caffeine stresses your heart by making it pump faster, and it also raises triglycerides, a form of fat in the blood that increases risk of heart attack. Many experts advise people who have heart disease against having coffee and other caffeinated beverages. But don't depend on decaf to take their place. The oils in decaffeinated coffee actually raise LDL levels more than regular brew does, says David Jenkins, M.D., Ph.D., professor of medicine and nutritional sciences at the University of Toronto.

GET INTO GRAPES. The alcohol in wine helps protect against heart disease by raising HDL cholesterol. But that's not where it ends: There's an LDL-lowering compound in grape skins, says Leroy Creasy, Ph.D., of Cornell University College of Agriculture and Life Sciences in Ithaca, New York. So even if you're not into wine, you can still protect against heart attack by eating grapes or drinking grape juice.

HAVE AN APPLE A DAY. Apples contain antioxidant compounds called flavonoids that damage LDL cholesterol and keep it from sticking to artery walls. Flavonoids are found in 4,000-plus different foods (including garlic and onions), but flavonoid-rich apples get a lion's share of research attention. In a five-year study in the Netherlands, researchers found that people who ate an apple a day along with some other flavonoid-rich foods had one-third the heart attack risk of those who didn't eat these foods.

....

Immune Function
Beta-Carotene and Other Immunity Boosters

ONE "AH-CHOO!" FROM A CO-WORKER, and a drifting cloud of viruses swarms through the air. Bacteria and fungi clandestinely attack our bodies through our noses, mouths or skin. Various parasites that we consume in food and water harm our intestinal tract, lungs, liver or brain. Even pollutants and toxins in air and water weaken our immunity and trigger life-threatening diseases.

Any one of these microscopic menaces can cause an infection or trigger a disease. Yet each day our bodies must do battle with untold billions of them—over one million bacteria can live on a single inch of freshly washed skin.

A strong immune system can not only wipe out these invaders before they can cause illness but can also help prevent and control serious conditions such as cancer. There's even research that indicates that a strong immune system can delay the onset of AIDS in those infected with HIV.

The problem is, immunity tends to weaken with each passing year. "As you age and reach your fifties and sixties, your immune system changes," says Ronald Watson, Ph.D., research professor at the University of Arizona College of Medicine in Tucson. "Your infection-fighting cells don't function as well, placing you at greater risk for infection and cancer."

Your body fights constant battles with its invaders. "I hate to use military terminology, but it's really war going on inside your body between these infectors and your immune system," adds Terry Phillips, Ph.D., D.Sc., director of the immunogenetics and immunochemistry labs at George Washington University Medical Center in Washington, D.C., and co-author of *Winning the War Within: Understanding, Protecting and Building Your Body's Immunity*. "If you think of your body as being a country, the immune system is the army—attacking these invaders to keep the peace."

And as Napoleon said, "An army marches on its stomach." Or at least, scientists may add, the right diet can keep it strong. "The immune system is like every other system in the human body: It requires a healthy diet in order to function properly," says Dr. Phillips. "And certain nutrients have been shown to boost your immune system's response and make you more resistant to disease. Besides that, the right diet gives you the energy you need so you can exercise—which also keeps immunity strong—and ensures that you get the proper sleep so your immune system gets a chance to repair itself."

Meet the Megavitamins

Leading the "Most Wanted" list of immunity-boosting vitamins are vitamin C, vitamin E and beta-carotene. These antioxidants help build immunity for the same reasons they protect against cancer and keep you looking and feeling younger.

"An antioxidant is anything that scavenges free radicals (unstable molecules that harm cells and tissues) and protects against oxidative damage," says Harinder S. Garewal, M.D., Ph.D., assistant director of cancer prevention and control, section of hematology-oncology at the Veterans Administration Hospital and the Arizona Cancer Center, both in Tucson, Arizona, who pioneered the study of beta-carotene as a possible way of decreasing cancer risk.

In a review of more than 200 studies conducted over a 20-year period, the Alliance for Aging Research—a Washington, D.C.–based public health organization—concluded that vitamins C and E and beta-carotene do help squelch free radicals. While scientific researchers have not agreed on specific recommendations, they do suggest getting more antioxidant vitamins in your food. Here's how.

EAT CITRUS FRUITS. "Citrus fruits like oranges and grapefruit are among the best sources of vitamin C," says Dr. Phillips. You'll get even more vitamin C in tropical fruits such as guavas, papaya and kiwifruit than you get from an orange.

NIBBLE NUTS AND SEEDS. Almonds, other nuts and sunflower seeds are among the best food sources of vitamin E. Actually, you'll get more vitamin E from cooking oils than anything else, but easy does it: Even "healthy" oils get all their calories from fat and can add extra pounds.

"Vitamin E is an inhibitor of free radicals, and it's also supposed to be good for red blood cells," says Dr. Phillips. "It also helps boost immunity by stimulating B and T cells."

EAT YOUR VEGGIES. The best sources of beta-carotene are fruits and vegetables that have an orange or yellow color, such as squash, mangoes and carrots, as well as green leafy vegetables such as spinach and kale. "Beta-carotene stimulates the natural killer cells' activity and has an overall positive effect on immunity," says Dr. Garewal.

Low Fat, High Immunity

The link may be better established in heart disease, cancer and scores of other illnesses, but research seems to indicate that dietary fat may also worsen an innocent cold or slow the healing of wounds. "There is no question that a low-fat diet is important for strong immunity," says William Adler, M.D., chief of medical immunology at the National Institute on Aging in Bethesda, Maryland.

Various studies by scientists at the U.S. Department of Agriculture Western Human Nutrition Research Center in San Francisco reveal that the more fat in your diet, the less effective your immune system. "All things being equal, the less fat you eat, the stronger your immunity to disease," says Darshan Kelley, Ph.D., research leader of these studies.

The problem is that many of the foods that help build immunity, such as meat, are also high in fat. Here's how to get the nutrition you need for a top-notch immune system without having to go to the last notch on your belt.

DON'T GO OVERBOARD. "Very low fat diets don't taste very good, so it's very unlikely that you'll stay on them very long," says Dr. Adler. His advice: Try to get between 20 and 30 percent of your total calories from fat sources. This is in contrast to the typical 40 percent in the American diet. "This can be accomplished fairly easily, simply by watching your intake of animal sources like fatty meats, ice cream and butter," he says.

LIMIT YOUR CONSUMPTION OF MEAT. Try to limit animal sources—even lean ones—to one three-ounce serving two or three times a week. But there's no need to give up meat altogether if you haven't already. "Fish and lean meats like chicken contain a lot of nutrients, so don't feel as though you have to avoid them entirely," says Dr. Adler.

GO FOR THE PRODUCE. "The best way to get the nutrients you need for strong immunity without a lot of fat is to make fresh fruits and vegetables the focus of your diet," says James Hebert, Sc.D., associate professor of medicine and epidemiology at the University of Massachusetts Medical School in Worcester. There are a few exceptions, such as coconuts, that are high in fat, "but generally, a diet rich in fruits and vegetables will give you what you need for stronger immunity," says Dr. Hebert.

EAT WITH THE SEASONS. One way to keep a fruits-and-veggies diet interesting, says Dr. Adler, is to follow the seasons of freshness. "By following the seasons, you become more educated to freshness and, as a result, enjoy eating produce more. Buy apples in autumn and peaches in summer—whatever is in season. That way you'll get the best tastes at the best time."

LOSE THE BOOZE. Alcohol seems to impair the immune system. "Even occasional drinking may displace certain key nutrients—especially the antioxidant and B vitamins," says Ronald Watson, Ph.D., research professor at the University of Arizona College of Medicine in Tucson. "Moderate or heavy drinking definitely reduces the absorption of these vitamins and suppresses the immune system." That means that you'd have to eat more foods rich in these key nutrients in order to keep your immune system from suffering.

The Zinc Link

"You hear a lot about the antioxidant vitamins, which protect against damage done by oxidation—a process that can weaken immunity," says Dr. Phillips. "But they're only part of the story. In fact, there are other nutrients that may be just as important—or even more so—in keeping immunity strong."

Leading the list is zinc, an often overlooked and under-appreciated mineral best known for helping heal wounds and build tissues. "It may also be the single most important key to a healthy immune system," says Dr. Phillips.

Zinc helps build T cells, the front-line defense in a strong immune system. Studies show that people deficient in zinc are more prone to infection and overall immunity weakness.

Research has also found that people with immune system problems may be able to correct such problems if they take zinc supplements, according to zinc researcher Ananda Prasad, M.D., Ph.D., professor of medicine at Wayne State University School of Medicine in Detroit. But even if you don't have a deficiency problem, it does your body good to make sure it has an adequate zinc supply. Among the foods that are high in zinc and can help you be more resistant to disease are meat and potatoes.

For both men and women, the recommended level, or Daily Value (DV), for zinc is 15 milligrams per day. Women, however, should get up to 20 milligrams per day during their childbearing years, according to Dr. Prasad. "Unfortunately, most people only get about half that amount—between 8 and 10 milligrams," says Dr. Prasad. If you get a lot of fiber in your diet and very little meat, you may be running a zinc deficit, according to Dr. Prasad. (Your doctor will be able to tell you if there's a problem.) But for many other health conditions—such as high cholesterol and high blood pressure—a high-fiber, low-fat diet is recommended.

So what tactics can you use to make sure that you boost your zinc without clogging your arteries? Read on for some answers.

EAT OYSTERS. A half-dozen medium oysters contains over

75 milligrams of zinc. In fact, just one oyster provides close to your entire daily requirement.

CONSUME MEAT OCCASIONALLY. You may be trying to cut down the amount of meat you eat in order to reduce the fat in your diet, but don't cut it out completely. "In moderation, red meats are fine—even for people trying to reduce the fat in their diets," says Dr. Phillips. Just choose lean cuts of red meat such as beef top round—which has about five milligrams of zinc and four grams of fat per serving. And if you're not into red meat, chicken and turkey are also fine sources of zinc.

Nonmeat sources of zinc include eggs, whole grains, wheat germ, potatoes, pumpkin seeds, green beans and legumes such as lima beans and peas.

WATCH YOUR IRON INTAKE. Zinc and iron have something of a seesaw relationship, says Dr. Prasad. "Iron and zinc interfere with the absorption of each other. In particular, iron supplements interfere with zinc absorption, making that mineral unavailable to your body." There is no way around this—you need iron for strong immunity. But this can mean trouble for menstruating women, who lose iron during menstrual bleeding. In fact, they may require iron supplements to keep from becoming anemic.

"I guess the best advice is that if you're a woman taking iron supplements, realize that you need to eat more foods rich in zinc," says Dr. Prasad. (Men rarely need iron supplements because they usually get enough iron in their diets.)

More Immunity-Boosting Minerals

Some essential minerals can give you the protection you need against infections and disease—particularly as you age. What's more, a little goes a long way. "Usually, there's no need to take supplements for these minerals," says Dr. Prasad. "A good diet is usually enough to supply you with what you need."

Iron. This mineral helps carry oxygen to all cells—including immune cells that engulf invading bacteria and kill them with a deadly chemical. If you have low levels of iron, you might be more susceptible to bacterial infections, especially in your intestinal tract. Low iron can also make you more prone to viruses since defenses are weakened by lack of this mineral. The DV for iron has been set at 18 milligrams per day for both men and women. Although meat is often thought of as the primary source of iron, there's also abundant iron in beans, nuts, seeds and tofu.

They Serve and Protect

Food is needed for the care and feeding of the billions of new cells produced in your body each day. Since most of these cells live only a few days, they constantly need to be replaced. Among these cells are the warriors that comprise your immune system. These guardians of your body protect you from what are generally called antigens—the term used for anything thought to be an invader, such as viruses, bacteria, dust or chemicals. Your body protectors include:

Antibodies. These Y-shaped protein molecules rush to the infection site, neutralizing the enemy with a chemical or tagging it for attack by other cells.

Killer T cells. These cells are so named because they mature in the thymus, a lymph gland that sits behind the breastbone. Killer T cells do the dirty work—specializing in killing cells that have been invaded by foreign organisms such as viruses, bacteria and other attackers. They also destroy cells that have become cancerous.

Helper T cells. These do-gooders actually identify the antigen and then call in the reinforcements—which are usually killer T cells.

Suppressor T cells. These specialized cells assist helper cells in mobilizing the fighting force. But their main job is to call off the troops once the infection has been conquered.

Selenium. By activating the infection-fighting troops in your immune system's army, selenium prevents oxidative damage to cells. It also boosts the immune system function of vitamin E and prevents cancerous tumors. Though there is no DV for selenium, many nutritionists recommend that you get at least 70 micrograms every day—the amount you'd get from

B cells. These brutes function like arms dealers. Formed in bone marrow, they deploy the weapons—the powerful chemicals used by your antibodies and your T cells to destroy the enemy. B cells also carry the "memory" of previous battles with specific antigens. Essentially, they keep records of previous battles so that any repeat invasion by a former foe can be immediately countered. When the T cells are called up as reinforcements, the B cells often enter the fray with them.

Macrophages. These are big cells that move slowly through the bloodstream looking for any signs of trouble. When they find an antigen, they turn into monstrous gluttons that engulf and eat it. Macrophages also summon helper T cells to the scene.

Neutrophils. These are the search-and-destroy team of the immune system. These cells are faster-moving than macrophages, which ooze amoeba-like through cells in your blood vessels. A neutrophil flows around its prey, enveloping it and then destroying it with enzymes.

It's a highly specialized system, with each cell having a specific role. But you're the one who feeds the troops. And when you eat the right diet, you help them do their jobs.

half a tuna sandwich. Selenium is found in virtually every food, with highest amounts coming from fish, shellfish and whole grains.

Magnesium. This mineral helps make infection-fighting white blood cells. Fall short on this nutrient and your immune system can become overstimulated and aggressive, with immune cells attacking and damaging the body. Both men and women need about 400 milligrams a day of magnesium. You'd get that from a couple of handfuls of sesame seeds. Certain prescription drugs can deplete magnesium stores, so check with your doctor about this if you're taking long-term medication. Drinking alcohol can also deplete magnesium.

Copper. Copper helps keep the immune system working hard when it's fighting infection. A deficiency in copper may lead to a lower white blood cell count and less resistance to infections. And if you don't have enough copper, cells that kill dangerous bacteria or viruses may become less active. Veal and lamb liver are good sources of copper, but these organ meats are high in cholesterol. Next best are oysters. At the first sign of a cold, doctors say, it might be wise to increase copper intake slightly.

A Major Role for Micronutrients

The ideal diet for building immunity is the same as a prescription for healthful eating. "Probably the best diet for immunity is one that's low in fat and contains all the major nutritional components—proteins, carbohydrates and even a little fat," says Dr. Phillips. "But one of the most overlooked—and important—aspects of eating for stronger immunity is to get plenty of the 'micro' nutrients that everybody has to worry about but nobody ever does," he adds. He points out that there are many lesser-known vitamins and minerals that also help nourish the immune system.

Here's how to get some of these other much-needed nutrients for strong immunity.

CHOOSE POULTRY. Chicken, turkey, goose and other fowl are great sources of vitamin B$_6$, which is crucial to strong immunity—especially as you age. "When older people were fed diets deficient in B$_6$, their immunity was lowered substantially," says Jeffrey Blumberg, Ph.D., associate director of the Jean Mayer USDA Human Nutrition Research Center on Aging at Tufts University in Boston. "When their intake was then increased one step at a time, immunity gradually returned to normal." Other good sources of B$_6$ include dark green, leafy vegetables (also a great source of immunity-building beta-carotene), bananas and prune juice.

FORTIFY WITH FOLATE. Good folate sources include dark green, leafy vegetables, eggs, legumes and salmon. (Liver is also high in folate, but it has too much fat and cholesterol.)

SELECT SELENIUM-RICH FOODS. This trace mineral is found—if only in the smallest amounts—in virtually every food we eat. Selenium, which like beta-carotene has antioxidant properties, is believed to activate infection-fighting cells and prevent oxidative damage to cells. Whole-grain cereals and breads are good sources, but expect a wide variance in the amount. (That's because selenium is in the soil, and different parts of the country have different amounts.) Selenium is also in animal products such as fish.

START THE DAY WITH MILK AND MAGNESIUM. Most ready-to-eat cereals are fortified with extra nutrients, giving you a lot of what you need for strong immunity—including magnesium, which keeps the immune system from becoming overstimulated and killing healthy cells. A bowl of shredded wheat with skim milk and a banana is an easy way to get over one-third of your daily quota for magnesium. Other good sources of this mineral include leafy vegetables, potatoes, whole grains and seafood.

When the Bugs Bite

There's little doubt that the right diet can make you more resistant to disease. But what should you do once a bug has bitten?

It depends on the ailment. Viruses respond better to food
(continued on page 152)

Sip Away the Sniffles

There's plenty of evidence to show that soups, teas and juices can actually help you get over your illness more quickly—and may even offer some added protection in preventing them. Here's an anti-sniffle smorgasbord.

HOT SOOTHERS—A DIFFERENT CUP 'O TEA

Any hot liquid helps cut congestion, says Frederick Ruben, M.D., professor of medicine at the University of Pittsburgh. When you drink something hot, it also raises the temperature in the throat, which slows viral reproduction. But these teas have an added bonus: They require no bags and contain no caffeine.

HOT LEMON TEA

Add 1 or 2 tablespoons lemon juice to 1 cup boiling water and stir in honey to taste.

PARSLEY TEA

Add 2 teaspoons dried parsley to 1 cup boiling water. Steep for 10 minutes. You can pour the tea through a strainer to take out the parsley.

SAGE TEA

Add 1 teaspoon dried sage leaves to 1 cup boiling water. Steep for 10 minutes and pour through a strainer to remove the leaves.

VINEGAR 'N' HONEY

Mix 1 tablespoon apple cider vinegar and 1 tablespoon honey in 1 cup hot water.

COLD QUENCHERS

Cool drinks help keep mucous membranes moist and prevent dehydration. Those high in vitamin C and other nutrients also replenish lost vitamins and feed your ailing immune system. Here are some of the best beverages for colds or flu.

CITRUS COMBO

In a pitcher, mix 2 cups grapefruit juice, 2 cups orange juice and ¼ cup lime juice. Serve over ice and garnish with mint sprigs. Makes four servings. (Per serving: 108 calories, 0.4 g. fat (3% of calories), 0 mg. cholesterol, 3 mg. sodium, 1.2 g. dietary fiber.)

ORANGE JUICY

In a blender, combine 1 can (6 ounces) thawed orange juice concentrate, 1 cup water, 1 cup milk, 2 tablespoons honey, 1 teaspoon vanilla and ⅛ teaspoon almond extract. Blend on high for 30 seconds. With the motor running, gradually drop in 4 cups ice cubes and blend until the mixture is smooth. Makes 4 servings. (Per serving: 138 calories, 0.2 g. fat (1% of calories), 1 mg. cholesterol, 35 mg. sodium, 0.3 g. dietary fiber.)

BANANA SMOOTHIE

In a blender, combine 2 medium bananas, 1 can (8 ounces) crushed pineapple (with juice), 1 cup crushed ice and ½ cup orange juice. Blend on high until smooth. Add 1 container (8 ounces) vanilla low-fat yogurt and process until blended. Makes 4 servings. (Per serving: 134 calories, 1.2 g. fat (7% of calories), 3 mg. cholesterol, 40 mg. sodium, 1.6 g. dietary fiber.)

than bacteria, which may require antibiotics. But here's some food for thought—or rather, recovery—the next time these common ailments start ailing you.

TAKE C. You probably know that vitamin C helps prevent and treat colds. What you may not know, however, is how much you should have when the sniffles start.

The answer: "Studies show that it takes about 500 milligrams to reduce sneezes and colds in cold sufferers," says Jeffrey Jahre, M.D., clinical assistant professor of medicine at Temple University School of Medicine in Philadelphia and chief of the Infectious Disease Section at St. Luke's Medical Center in Bethlehem, Pennsylvania. You'll get that amount in about five glasses of a vitamin C–rich juice, such as orange, pineapple, tomato or grapefruit, or in five oranges or large acerola cherries.

Mushrooms Show Their Magic

It's been over 2,000 years since Chinese herbalists first started using mushrooms to cure disease. Now Western doctors are discovering that this free-growing fungus may also help prevent it.

Several types of mushrooms—including shiitake and reishi—contain compounds called polysaccharides that boost immunity. Reishi mushrooms have also been shown to inhibit the development of cancer cells and reduce their number. In studies at the University of Texas Health Science Center in San Antonio, for example, reishi extracts were shown to have a significant anti-inflammatory effect. Other studies show that a diet rich in these mushrooms may help lessen problems associated with a variety of diseases ranging from arthritis to chronic fatigue syndrome.

Shiitake mushrooms, usually sold in dried form, are known for their firm texture and intense smoky flavor. If you get these mushrooms in dried form

TRY FIGHTING BRONCHITIS WITH HOT PEPPER. Another common virus, bronchitis, is known for producing some of the nastiest-looking phlegm you'll ever see. But eat spicy, and you can help bring an early end to this aggravating ailment. Foods such as hot peppers and curry help thin mucus, making it easier to cough up phlegm, says Varro Tyler, Ph.D., professor of pharmacognosy at Purdue University in West Lafayette, Indiana, who has done extensive research on the use of herbs and traditional remedies.

In fact, spicy foods are good for any kind of congestion, including a stuffy nose. The general rule: If it makes your eyes water, it will do the same *inside* your body.

CLEAR UP COLD SORES WITH MILK. Cold sores (also known as fever blisters) come and go—usually during times of stress or when immunity is low—and usually occur on the

----

rather than fresh, they're easy to soften up for slicing. Simply soak them in boiling water for 15 to 20 minutes until they're soft and then slice them thinly. Shiitakes are available in many supermarkets, gourmet shops, farmers markets, health food stores and most Asian food markets.

Reishi mushrooms are not widely available and may have to be ordered through the mail. If they come dried, use the same soaking procedure to soften them up. If you get canned or fresh reishis, just slice them and add to any recipe calling for mushrooms. For more information about where to get both types of immunity-boosting mushrooms, contact the Alabama Shiitake Grower's Association, c/o Hosea Hall, Cooperative Extension Service, Alabama A & M University, Box 967, Normal, AL 35762 or Uncle John's Mushroom Company, P.O. Box 491, Doe Run Road, Unionville, PA 19375.

outside of your lips. They can also affect your nose, cheeks or fingers.

With an overall healthy diet you may be able to avoid these outbreaks, which usually last a week to ten days. But once they hit, applying whole milk (skim won't work) to the wound can speed recovery. Allow the milk to sit at room temperature before placing a compress directly on the wound, suggests Jerome Z. Litt, M.D., assistant professor of dermatology at Case Western Reserve University School of Medicine in Cleveland.

Also limit your intake of foods rich in arginine, an amino acid found in chocolate, cola, peas, cereals, peanuts, gelatin and beer. During outbreaks, avoid these foods altogether, since arginine "feeds" the herpes virus and may trigger cold sores.

TREAT CANKER SORES WITH YOGURT. "Eat at least four tablespoons of unflavored yogurt every day, and you'll prevent canker sores," advises Dr. Litt. It's believed that the beneficial bacteria in live-culture yogurt zap canker sores, which seem to strike during times of stress, when resistance is lowered. (If the yogurt contains live cultures, the label will say so.)

Other experts say that you may be able to avoid canker sores by eating more vitamin C–rich foods, such as broccoli, cantaloupe and red peppers. Stay away from acidic vitamin C foods like citrus fruits while you have a canker sore, though, because the irritation from acidity will cause you more pain.

TO DITCH YEAST INFECTIONS, AVOID SUGAR. Yogurt is one way of handling this common form of vaginitis; the active cultures fight the *Candida albicans* virus, the culprit behind yeast infections. A diet rich in vitamin C is also advised.

But if you're prone to common and stubborn yeast infections, try to rein in your sweet tooth. Sugar can cause chronic yeast infections, says Jack Galloway, M.D., clinical professor of obstetrics and gynecology at the University of Southern California School of Medicine in Los Angeles. Brown sugar and honey seem to cause fewer problems than white sugar, but it's still a good idea to limit your intake of sweets.

Irritable Bowel Syndrome
Colon-Calming Strategies

TALK ABOUT A STORMY MONDAY! First your annual performance review, then a hurried lunch and then a bout of diarrhea. It got worse: Tuesday brought crampy gas pains, and Friday found you constipated. If you're among the estimated 36 million American women with irritable bowel syndrome (IBS), you know that your bowel can move in mysterious and inconvenient ways. Irritable bowel syndrome may be a chronic or recurrent disorder—symptoms may include bouts of diarrhea with pain, gas and sometimes constipation. So far, no one knows what causes it.

And sometimes food and stress seem to spark the symptoms of IBS—so much so that some women avoid certain foods altogether, leaving them vulnerable to nutritional deficiencies. Yet there's reassuring news about diet and IBS—doctors say the right food choices can help control your symptoms.

"IBS is not life-threatening, but it can be a nuisance for some women and a life-altering experience for others," says Roger Gebhard, M.D., professor of medicine at the University of Minnesota in Minneapolis and staff physician at the Minneapolis Veterans Administration Hospital. "No one really knows what causes these abnormal spasms in the small intestine and colon. It may seem that certain foods can set things off, and so can anxiety or tension or an important deadline at work."

We all get a touch of diarrhea, irregularity or a tummy ache once in awhile. But you may have IBS—and should see a doctor—if you experience abdominal distress daily or intermittently for at least three months and your bowel movements seem to be an on-again, off-again affair at times. Pay attention to changing stool frequency, changes in stool consistency (from watery to hard, for example), excessive straining, passage of mucous and abdominal bloating.

"The first thing we look at is the relationship between your diet and how you're feeling," says Charlene Prather, M.D., senior associate in the Department of Internal Medicine, Division of Gastroenterology at the Mayo Clinic in Rochester, Minnesota. "Just removing certain foods or adding others can work wonders."

IBS is tough to "cure." If dietary strategies bring only limited relief, doctors sometimes recommend over-the-counter medications containing loperamide for diarrhea, dietary fiber supplements to relieve constipation and prescription spasm-stopping medicines to block the clutching aches that many people with IBS feel after eating. Relaxation exercises are often part of the treatment, too.

Uncover Your Mealtime Land Mines

Where to start? That depends on whether your biggest IBS complaint is diarrhea, pain or constipation, says Dr. Prather, so pay attention. At the first sense of pain or diarrhea, try to remember what you ate last. The usual culprits include (but aren't limited to) sugar-free candies and cookies containing sorbitol and antacids containing magnesium. If you're lactose intolerant (that means you lack the enzyme that digests milk sugars), milk products could cause a stir. Did you have a cappuccino? Caffeine and fat can stimulate your colon, making it move uncomfortably fast. Beer and tacos? Alcohol and spicy foods may rile things up, as can carbonated drinks.

For some people, certain carbohydrates seem to be problematic, says Dr. Prather. Beans, broccoli, cauliflower, apples and other fruits and vegetables—even salads and forms of bran—can cause cramping and diarrhea.

"There are about 20 different kinds of carbohydrates that some people digest poorly, leaving them with gas and loose stools, even if the food is natural. A patient of mine was drinking a gallon of apple juice a day, for example. Once she stopped, her symptoms cleared up. For other people, the problem food might be mushrooms, or even lettuce. It's very individual," Dr. Prather says.

Don't Gulp and Go

How, when and where you eat can be as important to a restful bowel as what you eat, says Charlene Prather, M.D., senior associate in the Department of Internal Medicine, Division of Gastroenterology at the Mayo Clinic in Rochester, Minnesota. "Mealtime stress can trigger bowel contractions and spasms that cause problems. Also, when people eat too quickly or are anxious while eating, it increases air swallowing, which can make you feel bloated and give you gas," adds Dr. Prather.

So don't mix mealtime with business.

"I always advise people with irritable bowel syndrome—and everyone else, for that matter—to devote their lunch breaks to lunch and nothing but lunch," notes Elizabeth Ward, R.D., a nutrition counselor with the Harvard Community Health Plan in Boston. "Don't chow down on a sandwich and then run ten errands. You need time to relax."

The same goes for breakfast and dinner. *Slow down.* And save animated conversations for later. Talking a lot while eating may also cause excess air-swallowing, says Barry Jaffin, M.D., a specialist in gastrointestinal motility disorders and clinical instructor in the Department of Gastroenterology at Mount Sinai Medical Center in New York City. "Bolting your food or talking at the same time can be long-standing habits that are hard to break," he says. "Changing may take a little time."

If you're not absolutely certain that you've nabbed a culprit, you might try eating *more* of that food and note the results, Dr. Gebhard suggests. If it bothers you, you'll know it.

Keeping Things Calm

Obviously, if you've made a clear connection between IBS and certain foods, you should stop eating the foods that provoke symptoms, says Dr. Prather. Here's what else experts suggest.

EAT LEAN. Fat is the strongest dietary stimulant of intestinal contractions. Trim all visible fat from meat, switch to non-fat dairy products and use butter, margarine and oil sparingly.

"Fat will stimulate a hormone that can cause contractions of the bowel," says Barry Jaffin, M.D., a specialist in gastrointestinal motility disorders and clinical instructor in the Department of Gastroenterology at Mount Sinai Medical Center in New York City. "If you decrease fat intake, it may decrease the contracting hormones. I'll tell a patient with pain-predominant IBS to try that."

INTRODUCE YOURSELF TO FIBER—GINGERLY. If constipation's got you all clogged up, you may need more fiber and fluids in your diet, says Dr. Gebhard. One caveat: If you have IBS, you may have to add fiber more slowly, he says.

"Start with a small amount and build up," he suggests. "Fiber is a balancing act. Add too much too fast, and you can get bloating, gas or pain. Increasing your intake slowly is less likely to make you uncomfortable."

How slowly? Dr. Prather suggests adding 5 grams a day (about the amount in a half-cup of high-fiber cereal) for one week. Every week, add another 5 grams a day until you're consuming 20 to 35 grams a day.

DRINK LEMONADE—OR OTHER FLUIDS. "I ask women to please make sure they get a minimum of eight 8-ounce glasses a day of water, juice, lemonade, skim milk or herbal tea," adds Dr. Prather. "You need plenty of liquids so the fiber bulks up and moves stools more quickly through your bowels. Otherwise, the fiber just sits there and makes matters worse."

(For additional tips on adding more fruit, vegetables and whole grains to your menu, see "Constipation" on page 93.)

DIVIDE AND CONQUER. Overeating stretches your lower gastrointestinal tract—and it's the stretching that causes pain, says Dr. Prather. "So skipping breakfast and lunch and eating a huge dinner is not a good idea. Spread your intake throughout the day."

If even regular-size meals leave you in agony, try four or five mini-meals spaced throughout the day instead of three main meals, says Elizabeth Ward, R.D., a nutrition counselor with the Harvard Community Health Plan in Boston. "Plan ahead and include fruit, vegetables, whole grains, protein—everything you'd normally eat—redistributed. And focus on good nutrition—a doughnut and a cup of coffee won't do it," she adds.

....

Jet Lag
Don't Let Air Travel Drag You Down

THE MODERN JET GETS US where we're going so quickly that we think nothing of taking a long weekend several time zones away from home. If it's a pleasure trip, you want to enjoy it; if you're on business, you want to be sharp and think clearly. It doesn't matter whether you lose a couple of days readjusting to the time change if you're going to be away for several weeks, but if your total time budget is only three or four days, you don't want to spend it feeling like a zombie, regardless of your mission.

The human body has a rhythm to most of its functions. We are programmed to sleep when it's dark and awaken when the sun comes up; our temperature is higher every evening than it is in the morning. These patterns all reflect "circadian rhythm," the intricate, programmed ebb and flow of our hormones. When you board a jet in New York City at 7:00 P.M., the clock will read 7:00 or 8:00 A.M. some seven hours later when you arrive in Europe because of a five- or six-hour time difference. However, as far as your body is concerned, it's still 2:00 A.M. While you're flying, sitting for hours in a space meant for a five-year-old, your biological timekeeper keeps going. By the time you arrive in the early morning, you're ready for bed. But you haven't spent all that money to be holed up in a foreign hotel, so you drag yourself about, convinced that you're having a good time. That enervation lasts two or three days and is what we call jet lag. No sooner do you begin to adjust to the new time than you're on your way home, and the process starts again at the other end.

Feast, Fast and Feast Again

Scientists have been trying for years to develop drugs and chemicals to fool the body into thinking night is day and day is night. A breakthrough may finally be in the offing in the form of melatonin, a natural body hormone. Until its proper dosage is determined, you can ease the symptoms of jet lag by modifying what and when you eat as you prepare for your trip across several time zones. Here's how to do it.

First, fly during the day whenever possible. That's not always easy, because London and Paris are currently the only European destinations to which you can fly in the daytime from the United States. These flights leave around 10:00 A.M. Eastern time (that's 3:00 or 4:00 P.M. in Europe). You arrive in the evening after a six- or seven-hour flight. By the time you've collected your baggage, completed the airport formalities and reached your hotel in town, it's bedtime. Perfect! You'll have a good night's sleep, and the next morning you should be able to start the day feeling fairly fresh. You may peter out somewhat earlier than usual, but there is not too much jet lag on this kind of schedule.

Also, try the feast-fast-feast dietary recommendations of the scientists at the Argonne National Laboratory (the research and basic sciences center of the U.S. Department of Energy).

It may help you to adapt to your biological rhythm more quickly. Here's how it's done.

For three or four days before you leave, get as much sleep as you can and avoid late nights. Three days before departure is a "feast" day, consisting of breakfast and lunch rich in

Eating to Ease Jet Lag

Want to try the jet lag diet? Here's a sample "fast" day.

FOOD	CALORIES
BREAKFAST	
⅓ medium cantaloupe	60
2 slices toast, light (40 calories per slice)	80
2 teaspoons low-sugar jelly	16
1 cup coffee or tea	5
LUNCH	
2 ounces tuna packed in water	70
1 tablespoon low-fat mayonnaise	50
2 slices bread, light (40 calories per slice)	80
1 medium apple	60
DINNER	
3½ ounces roasted chicken breast, skinless	173
1 small baked potato with skin	160
2 tablespoons fat-free dressing	20
½ cup steamed string beans	40
1¼ cups fresh strawberries	60
SNACK	
1 cup flavored sugar-free nonfat yogurt	100
TOTAL	**974**

protein—lots of fish, chicken, eggs (or egg white if you're on a low-cholesterol diet), turkey, nonfat yogurt or low-fat cottage cheese, high-protein cereals and beans. Dinner should consist mainly of carbohydrates—pasta, potatoes, starchy vegetables and sweet desserts (assuming, of course, you don't have diabetes). Also, and this is important, *do not have any caffeine between 3:00 and 5:00 P.M. on that day*. That means no caffeinated coffee, tea, cola, chocolate or cocoa. And watch out for the over-the-counter medications that contain caffeine. Check the labels to be sure. The most likely place you'll find it is in cough and cold remedies, to which the caffeine is added to counteract the drowsiness that these agents often induce.

The next day, that is, two days before you leave, is a "fast" day. Limit your intake to 800 to 1,000 calories, consisting of salads, clear soup, plain toast and fruit. To help reduce the number of calories, buy the 40-calorie-per-slice bread now widely available, use fat-free salad dressings and light fruit jellies and jams. Eat three servings of fresh fruit rather than just the juice to benefit from the bulk and fiber. Again, no caffeine in the afternoon. The sample menu on page 161 provides an example of a suitable "fast" day.

The day before departure is another feast day—same rules as day one.

The Day of Departure

On the day of departure you really do fast—nothing but water, of which you can have as much as you like. You may take whatever medications you normally would. If you're going west—toward the Orient from America or to Los Angeles from New York—eat *nothing* until 12:00 noon and no caffeine the rest of the day. If you're traveling east, for example, from Chicago to Paris, fast all day and drink no coffee or tea after 6:00 P.M. Try to sleep soon after you board the plane. Forget the movie, the food and any other distraction that the airline provides.

Once you're airborne, *drink no alcohol* whatsoever. Also, do not eat a full meal—stay with fruit, salad and cookies.

Dehydration is a common complication of long flights, so drink lots of mineral water or plain water.

What you eat the day you arrive is also very important. When it's breakfast time (regardless of whether you've arrived or are still on the plane), eat a high-protein breakfast. If you know that you will still be airborne at the time, order your breakfast ahead from the airline (you usually need to give a least one day's advance notice to order a special meal). Ask for a vegetarian meal and some low-fat cottage cheese. Eat your breakfast as close to 7:00 A.M. as possible and don't go back to sleep after you've finished. Read or walk around the plane.

After you arrive at your destination later that morning, assume the local mealtime schedule. Do not nap in the morning or afternoon, but retire early that evening.

Although most nutrition scientists are skeptical of all jet lag–fighting diets, some people feel that this feast-fast-feast regimen does help. Perhaps it's because of its effect on the enzymes that regulate the amount of sugar stored or released by the liver. In any event, it's worth trying. Bon voyage!

Kidney Stones
Shaking the Salt Habit May Roll Away the Stones

ROUGHLY 10 TO 20 PERCENT of men and 5 to 10 percent of women pass kidney stones sometime during their lifetime. About 80 to 90 percent of these stones are composed of calcium and oxalate. While it's been known for years that a high calcium concentration in the urine is one major risk factor, we also know that dietary calcium per se may not really be at fault. Now researchers may have uncovered one major—and unexpected—source of stone trouble, and it lives in your saltshaker.

Researchers analyzed urine concentrations among a group of 282 stone patients—one sample taken during a normal diet and one taken during a higher-than-normal-calcium diet (1,000 milligrams per day). What they found was surprising: Many of those on the normal diet had higher calcium concentrations in their urine (elevating stone risk) than those on the high-calcium diet.

Here's why: The patients with higher calcium concentrations in their urine also tended to have high sodium levels. "When your body tries to get rid of the excess sodium, it also excretes calcium—leading to a higher calcium concentration in urine and the higher risk for kidney stones," says endocrinologist William J. Burtis, M.D., associate professor of medicine at Yale University School of Medicine. "For patients at risk for these stones, sodium may turn out to be a more important risk factor than calcium itself." A smart move is to cut back on table salt and choose foods labeled "low sodium" when you shop. In the study, a low sodium intake was considered to be 2,500 milligrams per day; a high intake was 5,000 milligrams and above.

"People who are at risk should also get plenty of water to lower the calcium concentration in their urine even more," says Dr. Burtis. Eight glasses of water a day should cover your bases.

Menopause

Foods to Help You Keep Your Cool

HORMONE REPLACEMENT THERAPY, YES. But diet therapy to cool hot flashes and counter the potential health-robbing consequences of menopause? You probably won't find your doctor prescribing it. Yet those in the forefront of menopause research say that eating patterns may explain why women in many Asian cultures are less prone to hot flashes during menopause. Nor do these women appear to suffer the long-term aftereffects associated with dwindling estrogen levels: Asian women are far less prone to heart disease and hip fractures than Western women, for example.

Proof that diet can influence a woman's menopause experience is millions of research dollars away. Some researchers suspect, however, that the traditional Asian diet may hold an important key. Specifically, they have focused their attention on a diet that:

- Contains less than 20 percent of calories from fat.
- Restricts meat.
- Is rich in a variety of fruits, vegetables and whole grains, which are good sources of phytoestrogens.
- Includes at least one serving a day of tofu or some other soy food.

Wulf Utian, M.D., Ph.D., director of the Department of Reproductive Biology at Case Western Reserve University in Cleveland and executive director of the North American Menopause Society, describes this as an exciting area of study.

A plant-based diet, especially one that includes soy foods, is abundant in a group of natural chemical compounds called phytoestrogens, he explains. These compounds are converted in the gut to hormonelike substances that the body can mistake for estrogen.

Feeling Hot and Bothered? Avoid These Trigger Foods

Sizzling foods—either hot off a flame or fired with chili peppers—are notorious provocateurs. They can jack up your body temperature and send a red rush of heat through your face and chest. Alcohol and caffeine can likewise make you flush. It's best to avoid coffee, tea, cola and chocolate.

Phytoestrogens come in two general forms: isoflavones and lignins. Isoflavones are found primarily in soy foods such as tofu and soy milk; for lignins, the best sources that you can use are whole grains and flaxseed. Fruits and vegetables contain lignins, but in lesser amounts.

"We're not talking about large doses of these compounds," says Sherwood Gorbach, M.D., professor of community health at Tufts University School of Medicine in Boston and a leading phytoestrogen researcher. The Asian woman's diet averages about three to four ounces of soy foods a day, for example. That yields about 25 to 40 milligrams of isoflavones. In comparison, the average American woman eats at most only a few milligrams of isoflavones a day. Dr. Utian cautions, however, that foods containing phytoestrogens can be quite powerful and can have druglike properties. A serving or two a day of a soy food like tofu is a reasonable goal as part of a healthy, well-balanced diet. Because the role of dietary phytoestrogens in health is a new area of study, scientists are analyzing the various amounts of the compounds in various soy foods as well as the optimal level of intake.

Beyond this unique feature of many Asian diets, researchers point to the fact that, where Asian women age 50-plus enjoy robust good health, their diets contain little to no animal protein and are extremely low in fat, especially saturated fat.

In countries where the intake of protein—particularly animal protein—is low, there is a lower incidence of hip fractures compared with people in Western countries, according to Mark Messina, Ph.D., author of *The Simple Soybean and Your Health*. One reason may be that soy protein causes less calcium to be lost through urine.

After menopause, women no longer require as much iron as they once did. The Recommended Dietary Allowance dips from 15 milligrams to 10 milligrams after age 50, so one of the best reasons for eating meat—its bioavailable iron—is gone. Besides, compared with the leanest red meat, soy foods (which make good meat substitutes) are low in saturated fat. Only about 14 percent of the fat in most tofu is saturated. Low-fat

A Guide to Soy Foods

Look for soy products labeled "low-fat" or "fat-free," says dietitian Chavanne Hanson, R.D., of the University Hospitals of Cleveland. Many soy products are high in fat, so be selective. Note also the calcium levels, which can vary widely. Below are some values for the fat and calcium in certain soy products.

Note: Soft tofu is lower in fat than the firmer type because it contains more water—less whey has been drained off.

Some soy products like vegetarian or soy burgers are made with "soy-protein concentrate," which contains almost no isoflavones. If you see "soy-protein isolate" on the label, however, the isoflavones are largely retained.

SOY PRODUCT	FAT (g.)	CALCIUM (mg.)
TOFU (½ CUP; 4 TO 4½ OUNCES)		
Azumaya, soft	2.5	36.4
Azumaya, regular	3	221
Azumaya, extra firm	5	215
Mori-Nu, lite	1.3	26.6
Nasoya, soft	4	182
Nasoya, firm	6	189
Nasoya, extra firm	7	68
OTHER SOY FOODS		
1 cup Solait Instant Soy Beverage	3	300
1 ounce Soya Kaas soy cheese	5	15
½ cup defatted soy flour	0.6	121
½ cup cooked soybeans	8	88
1 Ken & Robert's Veggie Burger patty	2	0
½ cup tempeh	6.4	77

or light versions have even less. Certain brands also provide a decent dose of calcium. That's because some tofu is made by curding cooked, pureed soybeans with calcium compounds.

Of course at this point, the benefits to menopausal women of adopting an Asian diet as described here remain largely speculative. Nevertheless, many of the same dietary components have been cited by cancer experts as the key to cancer prevention. Following the "Sample Cancer-Shielding Menu" on page 84 may help keep cancer at bay and perhaps beat menopause's bad rap in the same bite.

....

Osteoporosis
Pack Your Bones with Protection

HAVE YOU HAD YOUR CALCIUM TODAY? To outsmart osteoporosis—the broken-bones epidemic that now hits half of all women over age 50 and an increasing number of men— the right diet with lots of calcium is crucial. That's true whether you're 25 or 65—it's never too soon or too late.

A save-your-bones diet is not as difficult as you might think. But it does take planning. Here's what it consists of.

- Eating three to four servings a day of foods listed in "Calcium Champs". These "white knights" provide a minimum of 300 milligrams of calcium per serving.
- Taking a multiple vitamin supplement containing 400 international units of vitamin D—to make sure that the calcium you consume gets absorbed.
- Limiting meat and sodium. Excesses of protein and salt cause calcium excretion.

How much of a difference will the right diet make? Top calcium expert Robert Heaney, M.D., professor of medicine at

Creighton University in Omaha, Nebraska, estimates that (combined with other good-diet strategies) getting enough calcium—the mineral that makes up most of our bones—could prevent as many as half of all osteoporotic fractures.

Too bad that surveys show most American women consume only about half the 1,000 to 1,500 milligrams of calcium they need daily. Men's diets, too, are falling short.

Calcium Champs

Choose from this list of winners to give your body a calcium boost.

ABOUT 500 MILLIGRAMS
- I cup Lactaid Calcium-Fortified Milk (lactose-reduced, nonfat)
- I serving instant breakfast drink made with nonfat milk

ABOUT 400 MILLIGRAMS
- I cup protein-fortified nonfat milk (available in some areas only)
- I cup plain nonfat or low-fat yogurt

ABOUT 300 MILLIGRAMS
- I cup flavored nonfat or low-fat yogurt (check label—some have less calcium)
- I cup nonfat or 1% low-fat milk
- I cup buttermilk
- I cup lactose-reduced nonfat or 1% low-fat milk
- 2 one-ounce slices nonfat or reduced-fat cheese
- I cup calcium-fortified orange juice
- I slice Wonder Calcium-Enriched Bread
- 2 slices Wonder Light Calcium-Enriched Bread
- I cup Solait Instant Soy Beverage
- I cup Rice Dream Enriched Beverage

Why don't we get enough? Maybe because it means working high-calcium foods into almost every meal. The good news: That isn't nearly as tough as many people think. Now that orange juice and bread come fortified with calcium, even milk-haters have smart options.

Make Calcium Champs Your Mainstays

To decide how many Calcium Champs you need, first find your daily calcium goal. Experts at the National Institutes of Health in Bethesda, Maryland, now advise women between

Calcium Contenders

You might not eat these high-calcium foods every day, but when you do, you're giving your body a calcium bonus.

ABOUT 300 MILLIGRAMS
- ½ cup evaporated skim milk
- I cup pudding from mix

ABOUT 200 MILLIGRAMS
- I cup nonfat or low-fat frozen yogurt, ice milk or ice cream
- ¼ cup nonfat ricotta cheese
- I frozen low-fat macaroni-and-cheese entrée
- I serving special calcium-fortified cereals

ABOUT 100 MILLIGRAMS
- ½ cup canned white beans
- ½ cup chopped cooked turnip greens
- ½ cup cooked shredded bok choy
- ½ cup chopped raw chicory (curly endive)
- I cup sherbet
- I ready-to-eat fat-free pudding
- 2 tablespoons instant nonfat milk powder

the ages of 25 and 50 and men between ages 25 and 65 to get 1,000 milligrams of calcium every day. Women over 50 and men over 65 need 1,500 milligrams; so do young adults under 25. (Pregnant or nursing mothers between 25 and 50 should add an extra 200 milligrams a day.)

Is your personal calcium goal 1,000 milligrams? Try to work three Calcium Champs into your diet every day. If your goal is 1,500 milligrams, aim for four Calcium Champs. With extra calcium from the rest of your diet and any multivitamin and mineral supplement you may take, you're certain to make the grade.

- 2 tablespoons nonfat cream cheese
- ¼ cup canned salmon with bones
- 2 canned sardines
- ½ cup low-fat tofu (check label—some have less calcium)
- 1 packet instant cocoa
- 1 tablespoon toasted sesame seeds
- 1 packet instant oatmeal

ABOUT 50 MILLIGRAMS
- ½ cup cooked broccoli
- ½ cup chopped cooked kale
- ½ cup canned kidney beans
- ½ cup canned pinto beans
- ½ cup cottage cheese
- 1 tablespoon grated Parmesan cheese
- 2 tablespoons nonfat sour cream
- 5 canned anchovies

Bonus Boosters for Strong Bones

Keep in mind the Calcium Contenders—high-calcium foods that you're not likely to eat every day: sardines, for example; or foods such as broccoli with a lower calcium content that doesn't add up very fast. That makes Contenders impractical to count in your daily quota. But do treat them as healthy extras to eat whenever you can!

Finally, if you simply can't work three or four Calcium Champs into your daily eating plan, make up the difference by taking calcium supplements, although calcium from food

A Bone-Saving Menu

Need some ideas to work more calcium into your diet? Give this sample menu a try.

FOOD	CALCIUM (mg.)
BREAKFAST	
1 cup whole-wheat flakes*	40
1 cup 1% low-fat milk	300
1 medium peach	5
MORNING SNACK	
1 cup calcium-fortified orange juice	300
1 large popcorn cake*	0
1 tablespoon peanut butter*	5
LUNCH	
1 cup bean soup	80
3 pieces sesame-rye crisp bread	0
2 one-ounce slices reduced-fat Cheddar cheese	300
AFTERNOON SNACK	
1 blueberry muffin	14

should always be your first choice. (Regular calcium intakes of up to 2,000 milligrams a day are safe for most people. If you have kidney stones, however, check with your doctor before taking calcium supplements.) To ensure a steady supply of vitamin D, some experts recommend a multi supplement with 100 percent of the Daily Value for vitamin D (400 international units). The only other major sources are milk (100 international units per cup) and sunlight acting on the skin. Studies show that many Americans get too little vitamin D. (But regular intakes should not exceed 800 international units per day.)

FOOD	CALCIUM (mg.)
DINNER	
1½ cups steamed Chinese vegetable mix*	86
1½ cups cooked brown rice*	30
13 medium cashews*	9
2 tablespoons sweet-and-sour sauce*	0
BEDTIME SNACK	
1 cup raspberry low-fat yogurt	350
TOTAL	**1,519**

NOTE: This menu also contains 1,799 calories with 48 g. fat (24% of calories). Add a multivitamin supplement with 400 IU vitamin D.

*For men, double the portion of these foods to reach 2,568 calories with 69 g. fat (24% of calories) and 1,689 mg. calcium.

Simple Ways to Get More Calcium

Want to crank up your calcium even further? Here are ten super-easy strategies to tuck more calcium into every meal.

1. "Cream" your cup of coffee with 3 teaspoons nonfat dry milk. Gain: 55 milligrams.
2. Stir ¼ cup nonfat dry milk into 1 cup nonfat milk. Gain: 220 milligrams, for a total of 520 milligrams. The taste is richer, too! Or buy fortified nonfat milk with about 400 milligrams per cup (you may have to hunt for this product; it's available in selected areas only).
3. Making puddings or "cream" soups? Use evaporated skim milk instead of regular nonfat milk. Gain: double the calcium.
4. Enjoy a cup of flavored nonfat or low-fat yogurt for dessert. Gain: 300 to 350 milligrams.

Give Your Bones a Nightcap

What's one of the best times for a high-calcium snack? Bedtime! A calcium nightcap may keep blood levels of calcium high enough overnight to stop calcium from being pulled out of your bones while you sleep. Here are two yummy recipes with serious calcium power.

Creamy Cocoa Cuddle. Prepare one packet reduced-calorie instant cocoa with ¾ cup evaporated skim milk instead of water. (587 milligrams calcium, 220 calories, less than 1 gram fat.)

Strawberry Dream. Mix 10 frozen strawberries, 1 cup strawberry nonfat yogurt, ¼ cup evaporated skim milk and a dash of vanilla extract in a blender until smooth. (486 milligrams calcium, 200 calories, less than 1 gram fat.)

5. Top a baked potato with ¼ cup nonfat sour cream. Gain: 80 milligrams.
6. Add 2 tablespoons Parmesan cheese to a pasta dish. Gain: 140 milligrams (3 grams of fat).
7. Slide a slice of nonfat cheese into your sandwich. Gain: 150 milligrams.
8. Spread 2 tablespoons nonfat cream cheese on your bagel. Gain: 80 milligrams.
9. Top 2 slices reduced-fat pizza with 5 anchovies. Gain: 50 milligrams (2 grams of fat).
10. Sprinkle 1 tablespoon toasted sesame seeds on a salad. Gain: 89 milligrams (4 grams of fat).

Important note: Remember that diet alone can't fight osteoporosis. Also essential are regular weight-bearing physical activity and, for many women, hormone replacement or other therapy after menopause. With these three major weapons, we give ourselves a fighting chance for bones that last as long as we do!

....

Ovarian Cancer
Adjust Your Diet, Reduce Your Risk?

IT USED TO BE YOU HAD to have a child or actively prevent one with oral contraceptives in order to lower your risk of ovarian cancer. But recent research shifts the focus from the kids to the kitchen. Findings suggest that ovarian cancer may also be thwarted with foods such as sugar snap peas and skim milk.

When researchers evaluated the eating habits of 450 women with ovarian cancer and 564 without, they saw that cutting ten grams of saturated fat a day (that's a switch from two glasses of whole milk to the same amount of skim) could trim the risk of ovarian cancer by 20 percent. And adding ten grams of vegetable fiber—what you'd find in about one cup of cooked lentils—may take down the risk another 37 percent. The study saw no relationship between unsaturated fats and risks for this cancer.

Small studies have hinted at links between diet and reduced risk of ovarian cancer, but this first, large study of the issues gives the idea some real weight.

"It appears possible to cut your risk of ovarian cancer in half by an aggressive modification of the diet," which would mean combining these behaviors, says Harvey A. Risch, M.D., Ph.D., associate professor of epidemiology and public health at Yale University School of Medicine.

Theories abound about how diet might affect hormones. Meat and dairy foods may contain small amounts of estrogen. Estrogen-like compounds are also found in vegetables. The brain may think they're the real hormone and halt its own production. Or the fiber in those vegetables may grab estrogen and escort it out of the body.

Of course the diet this study points toward isn't all that Spartan. Studies suggest that most people eat more saturated fat than they need to, and cutting it by a third by switching protein sources much of the time is a smart thing to do for other health benefits, too.

"The point isn't that people should never eat hamburgers," Dr. Risch says. "But things that are eaten regularly that are high in saturated fat should be cut back. People don't realize how little meat protein they need per day to live perfectly well. Four ounces of meat a day is probably sufficient for most women."

Pancreatitis
Eat to Beat a Bellyache

THE PANCREAS, SITUATED in the midline deep inside the belly, makes insulin and several enzymes that help digest food. Injury, inflammation and infection of this organ (pancreatitis) can be acute, lasting only a few days and followed by complete recovery, or it can become chronic, causing recurrent bellyaches every few weeks or months. The chronic form, which is often heralded by repeated attacks of acute pancreatitis, may lead to malabsorption of food and diabetes.

The number one cause of pancreatitis is drinking alcohol, especially more than 2½ ounces every day. People with acute pancreatitis often drink three or more times that amount.

One-third of all cases of acute pancreatitis are caused by

A Pancreas-Pacifying Plan

To help you plan your menus, here's a handy list of daily food servings, along with recommended fat and calorie contents, for people with pancreatitis.

FOOD	FAT (g.)	CALORIES
6 servings breads/grains/pasta	0	480
1 serving desserts, fat-free	0	200
4 servings fruits	0	240
2 teaspoons oil	10	90
4 ounces protein	12	200
2–3 cups skim milk	0	170–255
5 servings vegetables	0	125

gallstones passing from the gallbladder into the ducts and in-flaming the neighboring pancreas. A very high level of triglyc-erides (a neutral fat) in the blood can result in pancreatitis, too, presumably because this fat irritates the pancreatic cells. Also, since the pancreas lies directly behind the stomach, a peptic ulcer that doesn't heal can eat its way through the lining of the stomach and involve the pancreas. Some drugs, such as diuretics, tetracycline and estrogen can inflame the pancreas, as can viral infections such as mumps.

The result of pancreatitis is swelling of the ducts in the pancreas so that there is obstruction to the normal flow of the digestive enzymes to the intestine. The pancreas becomes en-gorged and its enzymes back up into its tissues, irritating and inflaming them.

The pain of pancreatitis—located in the middle of the upper abdomen and radiating through to the back—is excru-ciating and is usually accompanied by fever, nausea and vomit-ing. Sitting or leaning forward offers some relief. Unlike gallbladder pain, which comes in waves, this pain is steady and lasts for hours, even days.

Finding Relief

The dietary treatment of pancreatitis is simple but re-quires close medical supervision. Eat *nothing* during the acute phase. Most attacks are severe enough to require a stay in the hospital, where you'll receive all nutrition intravenously and have your fluids replenished. You'll get the painkillers you need, and when the attack is over, you'll be able to start drink-ing clear liquids, gradually returning to a normal diet.

If attacks keep recurring, more and more of your pancre-atic tissue will be damaged and its normal digestive functions progressively impaired. When that happens, much of the food you eat won't be sufficiently digested because of the lack of the necessary enzymes. The food will pass out through the stool almost intact. Digesting fat is the biggest problem. When the pancreatic enzymes are not available, the stool is loaded with fat, which has serious nutritional implications. Fat leaving the body in this way takes with it the fat-soluble vitamins (A, D, E and to some extent K), resulting in their deficiency.

If you have chronic pancreatitis, the most important single thing that you can do is stop drinking alcohol—completely and permanently. Some persons with chronic pancreatitis develop diabetes because the diseased pancreas cannot make enough insulin. They then usually require insulin or sugar-lowering drugs. The next step is to replace whatever enzymes the pancreas can no longer make. There are several of these enzymes on the market. Take one to three tablets before and during each meal or snack. Although the tablets go a long way toward replacing what's missing, it's not the same as having a normal pancreas. So challenge your pancreas as little

Do's and Don'ts to Soothe the Ache

Battling pancreatitis? Avoiding high-fat foods can help ward off episodes of irritation or inflammation.

Foods to avoid. Avocados; breads, waffles and croissants made with cheese and/or eggs; candy made with nuts, butter or cream; cream soups; cream vegetables; desserts such as cakes, cookies, ice cream, pastries and pies; doughnuts; egg yolks; fish packed in oil; meats such as bacon, beef, lunchmeats, sausage and veal; peanut butter; whole milk and whole-milk products such as butter, whole-milk cheeses, half-and-half, heavy cream, whipping cream and regular yogurt.

Acceptable options. Fat-free or light breads; hard candy; jelly beans; nonfat cereals; nonfat frozen desserts such as frozen yogurt and fruit ices; fruit gelatin; meringues; egg whites; fish, fresh or canned in water; jelly and jam; nonfat milk products such as nonfat cottage cheese, nonfat cheeses, nonfat yogurt and skim milk; pasta; soups such as defatted broth and fat-free vegetable soup; plain vegetables such as potatoes.

as possible with the food you eat, but be sure to get adequate nutrition. An upper limit of 15 percent of calories from fat, mostly from monounsaturated and polyunsaturated fats, is a realistic goal; you'll get animal fat in the protein allotment.

The enzymes that digest protein are also in short supply in chronic pancreatitis. As with fat, it will take a process of trial and error to see how much meat, poultry and fish you can handle comfortably. But you may want to consider limiting your animal protein intake to 25 to 30 grams daily, or three to four ounces of lean animal protein such as skinless chicken or fish. Animal protein provides the essential amino acids lacking in vegetable protein.

What does this leave you to eat? Lots of complex carbohydrates—vegetables, fruits, beans, pasta—prepared without added fat, the kind of diet that vegans follow. These foods do not require the pancreatic enzymes for digestion, so they must make up the bulk of your diet. Be sure to take a multivitamin containing the fat-soluble vitamins (A, D, E and K) as well as B_{12}, which is sometimes lacking in people with chronic pancreatitis.

"Do's and Don'ts to Soothe the Ache" on page 179 lists the foods to avoid and those you may eat if you have chronic pancreatitis. You're better off with several smaller meals than fewer larger ones. The table on page 177 is a guide to how much of each kind of food you should consume daily. It reflects a 15 percent fat content and 1,500 calories. If you need more calories, you may eat extra bread and fruit. If your triglyceride levels are very high, omit fruit juice and limit your intake of fresh fruit to two or three servings a day. Do not eat fat-free sugared desserts; eat those made with aspartame (NutraSweet) instead. Since it's not possible to get aspartame into baked desserts, you're likely to be eating the frozen variety. In short, this is the kind of diet prescribed for people with diabetes.

Can Antioxidants Calm a Troubled Pancreas?

There is an interesting twist to the management of pancreatitits—one that is still controversial, but promising.

Pancreatitis may be initiated or aggravated by free radicals, the end-products of many energy processes. These metabolic "bandits" are thought to contribute to most of mankind's health problems, ranging from the aging process to cancer to coronary heart disease.

Animal experiments have shown that when animals are pretreated with antioxidants—nutrients that neutralize free radicals, including beta-carotene, vitamin E and vitamin C—the degree of damage from pancreatitis is minimized. If you have pancreatitis, you may want to ask your doctor about taking antioxidants in supplement form.

In summary, chronic pancreatitis is usually the result of excessive alcohol intake or intolerance to it. In some cases, it is caused by gallstones or chemical substances or medications that damage the pancreas. Nutritional management consists of totally abstaining from alcohol, reducing your fat intake, decreasing the amount of protein you consume, eating mostly complex carbohydrates and replacing the missing pancreatic enzymes. Taking supplements of beta-carotene, vitamin E and vitamin C may also be helpful.

Premenstrual Syndrome
Eating to Ease the Discomfort

LIKE TAX SEASON, the *Sports Illustrated* swimsuit issue, widowed socks and inexplicable fashion fads, premenstrual syndrome (PMS) shows up with an unpleasant regularity.

With it come irritability, depression, insomnia, bloating, headaches, edginess, constipation, fatigue and breast tenderness—to name just a few pesky symptoms.

If that weren't enough, there's the out-of-control appetite and cravings for chocolate and chips that can accompany PMS—and seriously sabotage the best intentions to avoid fats, sugar, salt and other dietary goals. PMS can even exacerbate existing health problems such as asthma or allergies.

It's All in Your . . . Brain

Unfortunately, no one's sure why some women get PMS and others don't, or why some women have really distressing symptoms while others have mild ones. A lucky 15 percent of women actually report pleasant premenstrual side effects, such as an increased sex drive or creativity.

Levels of the sex hormones estrogen and progesterone fluctuate dramatically just before women menstruate. But that alone doesn't explain PMS. Studies show that women with the syndrome go through the same hormonal fluctuations that everyone else does. If hormonal fluctuations were the culprit, every woman who menstruates would have PMS.

Research suggests a more complex explanation. Women who get PMS may actually have a slightly different (but still normal) brain chemistry than those who don't. In these women, say theorists, the brain chemicals known as neurotransmitters that transmit messages through the nervous system may behave differently.

"For some reason their neurotransmitters respond differently to hormonal changes," says Andrea Rapkin, M.D., associate professor of obstetrics and gynecology at the University of California, Los Angeles.

Dr. Rapkin has found that women with PMS, for instance, produce lower levels of a feel-good neurotransmitter called serotonin than do women without PMS. A British study reports that deficiencies of other mood regulators, such as endorphins, could play a role in premenstrual distress.

Shortages of these chemicals or problems with the way the body uses them would explain some symptoms of PMS. Studies show that low levels of serotonin and other brain chemicals can cause depression and anxiety and trigger the kind of fat, sugar and salt combinations that many women report craving prior to their periods.

"There's a tendency for women to crave sweets and salty

foods premenstrually," says Jean Endicott, Ph.D., professor of clinical psychology in the Department of Psychiatry at the Columbia University College of Physicians and Surgeons and director of the Premenstrual Evaluation Unit at the Columbia Presbyterian Medical Center in New York City. "It may not always be chocolate; it could be pretzels or peanuts."

Studies suggest that these cravings could be the body's way of demanding a carbohydrate fix for a shortage of feel-good neurochemicals. When researchers at Massachusetts Institute of Technology in Cambridge fed women with PMS endorphin-boosting high carbohydrate meals, the women reported feeling less depressed, fatigued and tense.

Research has also shown that drugs capable of boosting serotonin activity eliminate some symptoms of the syndrome—suggesting that cravings could be an instinctive way of "self-medicating" with food.

A few studies suggest that calcium and magnesium, which play roles in the production of serotonin, may ease symptoms as well, notes James Penland, Ph.D., a research psychologist at the U.S. Department of Agriculture Human Nutrition Research Center in Grand Forks, North Dakota.

Is It Really PMS?

Chances are, if you have PMS, you know it. Usually, the telltale symptoms arrive a week to ten days before your period, disappear one to three days after it's begun, then come back to haunt you two weeks later.

Evidence indicates that as many as 95 percent of women have at least a few symptoms of PMS. Some experience the same symptoms in the middle of the month but notice that they worsen premenstrually. About 5 percent of women have symptoms so severe that they interfere with work and relationships.

Just to be sure that your symptoms are hormonally related and not caused by stress or psychological or medical problems—thyroid disorders cause similar symptoms—you need to keep a daily symptom diary for at least two months, says

Leslie Hartley Gise, M.D., associate clinical professor and director of the Premenstrual Syndrome Program at Mount Sinai School of Medicine of the City University of New York. Each day, note where you are in your menstrual cycle, what your symptoms are and their severity.

Also, think of yourself as a "food detective" and gather clues as to what might be causing your cravings. Does a Klondike bar soothe your jangled nerves? Does insomnia send you to the fridge for a bowl of cold spaghetti? Given the choice, would you opt for chocolate over sex? Look for a pattern, for symptoms appearing before your period but not during or right after.

Seven Symptom-Taming Tips

If you are suffering from PMS, a few changes in what you eat—and when—can help show symptoms the door.

EAT BEFORE A CRAVING STRIKES. Frequent, small meals high in complex carbohydrates can help you shake the moodiness and cravings that go with PMS, says Dr. Endicott. "Anecdotal evidence suggests that you're more irritable about four hours after your last meal," she explains. "So we suggest that women don't go more than three or four hours without eating something."

Make midmorning, midafternoon and after-dinner minimeals of fresh fruits and vegetables, says Dr. Endicott. Get creative. Put half a grapefruit under the broiler to bring out its sweetness. Freeze bananas, puree them in the blender, then refreeze the mixture in ice cube trays to make banana "ice cream." Slice a pear and pair it with tiny slivers of low-fat cheese. Spread spicy apple or pear butter on a toasted wholewheat English muffin.

BEWARE OF SUGAR-FAT COMBOS. As mentioned, studies suggest that women yearn for chocolate and other sweets before their periods because sugar and fat mixtures raise levels of the mood-lifting brain chemicals.

Unfortunately, sugary foods lift you up just to let you down, says Maria Simonson, Ph.D., director of the Health,

Weight and Stress Clinic at Johns Hopkins Medical Institutions in Baltimore. Eat a lot of sweets and your blood sugar will soar, then plummet, she explains. You end up feeling more dragged out than you did before the snack.

And if the sweets are both sugary and fatty, like chocolate cookies, you may also end up toting unwanted pounds.

Instead, reach for complex carbohydrate snacks, such as a toasted bagel or fresh vegetables dipped in hummus, suggests Joanne Curran-Celentano, R.D., Ph.D, associate professor of nutritional sciences at the University of New Hampshire in Durham. Or crunch some salt-free, whole-wheat pretzels or sweet cherry tomatoes. Those will keep your blood sugar, and energy level on an even keel, says Dr. Curran-Celentano. Your snack should not be eaten quickly, but should be savored and enjoyed, she says. You'll feel more relaxed and satisfied.

DRINK YOUR MILK. Research shows that women who get roughly 1,500 milligrams of calcium daily have fewer premenstrual symptoms than those who get 500 to 600 milligrams—the average day's intake for American women.

Shoot for at least 1,000 milligrams daily, advises Dr. Penland, preferably from calcium-rich foods, such as low-fat or nonfat milk, yogurt and cheese, collard and dandelion greens or canned salmon with the bones. If you miss the mark, he says, consider a calcium supplement.

LOOK FOR B$_6$. Like magnesium and calcium, vitamin B$_6$ seems to aid in production of serotonin, the feel-good brain chemical that may be in short supply in women with PMS, according to one study. A 100-milligram daily dose seems to help ease symptoms. Don't exceed that amount, though—high levels of B$_6$ can cause nerve damage. Try to get at least part of your daily quota from food. Bananas, turkey white meat, chicken breast, baked potatoes, chick-peas, spinach, tomatoes, brown rice, rainbow trout and fresh tuna are rich in B$_6$.

TOSS THE SALT. Salty foods can make water retention worse. If bloating is a problem, lose the saltshaker, says Dr. Rapkin. Try flavoring your food with herbs or a salt substitute such as Mrs. Dash. And avoid salty prepared foods.

(continued on page 188)

How Real Women Conquer Cravings

The women below shared their secrets for fighting PMS with food. Experts explain why these winning tactics work.

KELLY W., AGE 34

"I felt very depressed before every period. And I craved chocolate. Or I'd eat a whole bag of taco chips. I finally went to my gynecologist, and she recommended vitamin therapy. Now I take vitamin E, magnesium and B_6 when I feel the onset of symptoms. That eliminates the depression. I still have the food cravings. I try to eat unsalted pretzels—they're sugar-free and low in fat and sodium—or I eat just a little of whatever food I crave."

Why it works: Both B_6 and magnesium seem to aid the production of a feel-good brain chemical known as serotonin, low levels of which are associated with depression, according to a one study. As for snacking on pretzels, women who eat carbohydrates tend to report fewer feelings of depression and other mood disturbances associated with PMS, according to research at Massachusetts Institute of Technology in Cambridge. Salt contributes to water retention, says Andrea Rapkin, M.D., associate professor of obstetrics and gynecology at the University of California, Los Angeles, so unsalted pretzels are probably a good choice.

JANICE S., AGE 44

"I crave chocolate and sweets. So I suck on hard candy because that takes care of the sweet craving. And I allow myself a small cup of frozen yogurt in the evenings. That helps me get over the chocolate craving. I also double up on B vitamins, which helps keep me from being uptight and cranky. I take them two weeks beforehand. And I really try to watch my caffeine."

Why it works: Hard candy usually contains no fat; an ounce of milk chocolate has almost nine grams. So Janice is satisfying her sweet tooth while saving on unwanted fat. As for yogurt, women who get a hefty supply of calcium from dairy products such as yogurt suffer fewer PMS symptoms, says James Penland, Ph.D., a research psychologist at the U.S. Department of Agriculture Human Nutrition Research Center in Grand Forks, North Dakota.

And as Dr. Rapkin notes, B$_6$ seems to aid production of serotonin. Evidence indicates that caffeine, a stimulant in coffee and chocolate, may magnify premenstrual anxiety, says Jean Endicott, Ph.D., professor of clinical psychology in the Department of Psychiatry at the Columbia University College of Physicians and Surgeons and director of the Premenstrual Evaluation Unit at the Columbia Presbyterian Medical Center in New York City. So staying away from caffeine helps ease jitters.

KATHY S., AGE 33

"I have chocolate cravings. What works is not taking the first bite of chocolate. If I do, forget it. If I'm overwhelmed by the craving, I satisfy it with a low-fat McDonald's chocolate shake.

Why it works: Research done by neurobiologist Sarah Leibowitz, Ph.D., at Rockefeller University in New York City indicates that giving in to a craving for high-fat food tends to lead to cravings for more high-fat foods. So eating a low-fat version of whatever you crave helps keep PMS cravings under control.

"Some women find that they swell if they eat a lot of high-salt foods like pizza," Dr. Rapkin says. "If they already have swelling, it's reasonable not to eat those foods."

QUIT CAFFEINE. A mug of coffee may seem just the antidote to premenstrual fatigue. But it can cause more problems than it solves, says Dr. Endicott. There's some evidence that caffeine, a stimulant, will make you feel worse if you're anxious and irritable. It may also contribute to breast tenderness. So cut back on the coffee, tea, cola and chocolate, she suggests. But do it gradually. "Don't stop abruptly, because you are likely to get horrible headaches," she warns. Start drinking a brew that's three-quarters regular and one-quarter decaf. Move on to half regular and half decaf. Then graduate to all decaf.

DRINK IN MODERATION (IF AT ALL). Women who average ten or more alcoholic drinks a week are more likely to have moderate to severe PMS than nondrinkers, according to a study conducted at the Kaiser Permanente Medical Center in San Francisco, California.

Alcohol is also a depressant, so it'll make you feel worse if you're already blue, says Stephanie DeGraff Bender, clinical psychology director of the PMS Clinic in Boulder, Colorado. While dousing your spirits, alcohol will also lower your inhibitions, adds Dr. Endicott. And that's not necessarily beneficial.

"If you're angry, you're more apt to have an outburst if you've been drinking," Dr. Endicott says. "Angry outbursts, tearfulness and other impulsive actions may be facilitated by alcohol."

A Few More Do's

Dietary strategies against PMS are more likely to work if bolstered by other, nondietary strategies.

EXERCISE. Exercise can lift your mood, help you fight fatigue, relieve tension, make you more alert, help control your appetite and ease insomnia, according to the American College of Obstetricians and Gynecologists.

"It doesn't have to be aerobic dancing or in-line skating," Dr. Endicott says. "Twenty minutes of brisk walking helps.

Do it throughout the month, but particularly when you're premenstrual. Studies on fatigue show that, as a pick-me-up, 20 minutes of rapid walking is as beneficial as a 20-minute nap."

As a bonus, extra exercise will also help keep your weight stable if you tend to eat more before your period, Dr. Rapkin says.

QUIT SMOKING. The list of reasons to kick the habit keep growing. Here's another: Nicotine has a stimulating effect, but it wears off quickly, Dr. Gise warns, and you'll feel more fatigued than you did before you lit up.

TAKE TIME OUT TO RELAX. Stress can magnify the symptoms of PMS, Dr. Gise says. But some form of relaxation can help. When researchers taught women to relax with the help of guided imagery, complaints of premenstrual symptoms eased up considerably. Other options, including a few minutes of yoga or an exercise break, such as a walk around the park, may improve your outlook.

Skin Cancer
The Protective Effect of Going Low-Fat

FORGOING THAT BURGER and reaching for something less fatty might not only spare your heart and your scale. Recent research suggests that staying low in fat may also save your skin from precancerous changes.

Researchers halved the fat intake of 38 people with a history of precancerous skin lesions (called actinic keratoses), cutting it from 40 to 20 percent of the day's calories from fat. Another 38 people in the study continued their normal diets of 40 percent calories from fat. Two years later, there were only three new lesions in the low-fat group. There were ten among the group of 38 men and women who ate the same number of calories but didn't trim the fat.

"We may have shown that a low-fat diet does the same thing that sunscreens were shown to do in an earlier study—namely, prevent precancerous growths from arising," says study author John E. Wolf Jr., M.D., chair of the Department of Dermatology at Baylor College of Medicine in Houston. Not every skin cancer begins with a keratosis (and not every keratosis turns into cancer), but Dr. Wolf still sees the dietary route as an important skin-saving strategy. "If you're preventing precancerous growths, you're preventing some skin cancers," he says.

"Dietary manipulation may be helpful at any stage of your life," says Dr. Wolf. A low-fat diet may decrease the damage that's already occurred, he says, and that's important, since about 70 percent of sunlight damage occurs before age 17.

Fats seem to do their dirty work once they're broken down into different chemicals in the body, researchers theorize. A few of these chemicals have been associated with tumor growth in laboratory studies. Researchers also believe that fats act fairly late in the cancer-development process, at a stage called promotion and progression, rather than at the very beginning stage. It's possible that lowering the amount of fat in the diet right now could reduce these chemicals to a level less likely to produce cancerous changes, says Dr. Wolf.

This doesn't mean that you can take low-fat food on your hike and leave the sunscreen at home. But chopping out extra fat may fortify the skin cancer shelter that you've already built with sunscreen and protective clothing.

Weight Control
Fuel Up to Burn Fat

ONCE UPON A TIME, dieting meant simply cutting calories. We now know that this dieting strategy is like swimming up the Colorado River. You might make some progress, but ultimately, you're no match for nature.

For a diet strategy to succeed, it has to acknowledge the body's natural metabolic currents and flow with them. This food plan does. By following this simple formula, you'll maximize your body's natural fat-burning potential and peel pounds permanently. Specifically, the diet plan calls for:

- Eating four daily meals—breakfast, lunch, a substantial afternoon snack and dinner—each approximately the same size.
- Curbing fat intake while maintaining a moderate (not too low!) calorie intake.
- Focusing on naturally low-fat, high-fiber foods, such as vegetables, whole grains and legumes.
- Keeping a watchful eye on refined and processed foods that are calorie-dense and fiber-depleted.

Of course it's vital to add a heaping serving of exercise to any eating plan. Exercise activates weight loss; it revs metabolism so that you can eat enough calories to stay healthy.

The First Step to Weight-Loss Success

Spreading you daily calories over four meals is an effective way to speed the metabolism, minimize fat storage and dampen the appetite. Scientists have observed that missing meals, especially early in the day, is hazardous to the waistline.

"Skipping breakfast, eating a moderate lunch and a huge dinner is the most common pattern for people with weight problems," notes James J. Kenney, R.D., Ph.D., nutrition research specialist at the Pritikin Longevity Center in Santa Monica, California. Bypassing breakfast or lunch can result in overeating at dinner. And it can slow metabolism.

"We found that people who skipped breakfast, or breakfast and lunch, burned about 5 percent fewer calories than people who were eating three meals a day or more," says obesity expert C. Wayne Callaway, M.D., associate clinical professor of medicine at George Washington University in Washington, D.C. This pattern also affects production of the hormone insulin, which encourages fat production and storage, says Dr. Kenney. Large meals cause the body to release

Forewarned Is Forearmed

Before you find yourself with a bag of chocolate chip cookies in your lap with no clear recollection of how they got there, skim this list of potential danger zones.

At the supermarket: Never, ever shop on an empty stomach.

At mealtime: Preplan. "If you planned a healthy salad, you're more likely to follow through," says Georgia Kostas, R.D., director of nutrition at the Cooper Clinic in Dallas and author of *Balancing Act Nutrition and Weight Guide.* "If you didn't make plans, a hamburger will sound great."

After a meal: Pop a sugar-free mint or butterscotch candy into your mouth; resisting dessert will be easier.

At a restaurant: Order extra side dishes of rice and steamed vegetables. Eat more of those and less of the meat.

At a buffet party: After a few hors d'oeuvres, sneak off into the bathroom and brush your teeth.

more insulin. The time of day seems to make a difference, too: "In the evening the body responds better to insulin," says Dr. Kenney. "That means it stores fat more efficiently at dinnertime." The alternative—eating smaller, more frequent meals—not only reduces insulin but boosts the metabolism, burning more calories as well.

So a better plan would be to eat about 25 percent of your daily calories at breakfast and 25 percent at lunch. Add a substantial afternoon snack, also containing about 20 to 25 percent of your daily calories. (Research shows that small snacks—less than 10 percent of daily calories—don't raise the metabolic rate significantly.) Then eat a moderate dinner with about the same number of calories as your earlier meals. If you need an after-dinner snack, make it light and low-fat. If you've

---

You'll be less likely to eat more Swedish meatballs if they're going to taste like spearmint.

At the office: Visit the watercooler often or keep a carafe of water at your desk. Drinking eight glasses of water a day keeps you more satisfied and prevents overeating. A lot of people overeat from thirst, mistaking it for hunger, notes Kostas.

After dinner: Clean up the kitchen, turn off the lights and shut the kitchen down for the night so you don't have an excuse to keep going back for snacks, Kostas suggests.

In front of the TV: Put a thermos of ice water or hot tea on your TV table. Or lay out a preplanned healthy snack—like a measured amount of low-fat microwave popcorn.

On weekends: Make firm plans to eat every four to six hours. "If you're running errands and don't eat, the tendency is to get overly hungry and use your free time in a mall to grab high-calorie snacks instead of healthier choices," notes Kostas.

eaten well earlier in the day, you won't be as hungry for late-night munchies.

Calories Still Count

In determining your daily intake it's important to keep your eye on two horizons: fat and calories. While fat reduction

A Super Pound-Shedding Plan

Trying to lose a few? Give this low-fat, low-calorie menu a whirl.

FOOD	CALORIES	FAT (g.)
BREAKFAST		
¾ cup raisin bran cereal*	143	0.8
½ cup 1% low-fat milk*	50	1
1 whole orange in sections	65	0
½ pear	49	0
TOTAL	**307**	**1.8**
LUNCH		
1 cup lentil soup*	130	2.5
1 slice whole-wheat bread*	68	1.2
SALAD		
½ cup romaine lettuce	4	0
½ cup cucumbers	7	0
½ cup red peppers	14	0
2 tablespoons light ranch dressing	100	10
½ cup sugar-free chocolate pudding	92	2.7
TOTAL	**415**	**16.4**

is the most important priority for good health and weight loss, you don't want calories to fall too low or climb too high.

A good rule of thumb for women trying to lose extra weight is to eat 10 calories for every pound of your current weight; men's limit is about 12 calories. You can afford 2 to 3 additional calories per pound if you exercise for at least 30 minutes three times a week. This pace would result in a

FOOD	CALORIES	FAT (g.)
SNACK		
I cup low-fat fruit yogurt	240	3
½ cinnamon-raisin bagel*	100	0.8
I tablespoon low-fat cream cheese*	35	2.5
TOTAL	**375**	**6.3**
DINNER		
3 ounces swordfish*	132	4.4
MIXED VEGETABLES		
½ cup frozen peas	62	0
½ cup frozen carrots	26	0
½ cup brown rice*	110	1
½ mango	67	0
TOTAL	**397**	**5.4**
GRAND TOTAL	**1,494**	**29.9**

NOTE: This menu gets 18% of calories from fat.

*For men, double the portions of these foods to reach 2,262 calories with 44.1 g. fat (18% of calories).

half-pound to a pound a week weight loss, which studies show is the rate of weight loss that's most likely to be permanent and prevent the loss of valuable fat-burning muscle.

As for fat, most experts suggest about 20 to 25 percent of calories from fat. For best results, we recommend that calories from fat not exceed 20 percent of your daily calories—which is a ceiling of about 33 grams of fat for someone eating 1,500 calories a day, 40 grams for someone eating 1,800 calories, and 51 grams for someone eating 2,300 calories daily.

If you're uncertain how many fat grams or calories you're consuming, keep a food dairy for a couple of days. Then use a fat and calorie counter to find your totals. This is a winning technique. "Keeping records is consistently associated with

Five Ways to Curb Cravings

Why do dieters so often succumb to food cravings and binges? The most common trigger is undereating, says obesity expert C. Wayne Callaway, M.D., associate clinical professor of medicine at George Washington University in Washington, D.C. Overly restrictive diets set the stage for uncontrollable eating. Beyond that, here are some other experts' suggestions that should help keep bingeing at bay.

GO LOW-FAT, NOT FAT-FREE. Many people find that if they toe the fat-free line all day long, they never truly feel satisfied, says Georgia Kostas, R.D., director of nutrition at the Cooper Clinic in Dallas and author of *Balancing Act Nutrition and Weight Guide*. If hunger wells up soon after eating, try including some low-fat foods with each meal.

TRY TO "URGE SURF." When a craving strikes, resist momentarily; take a walk, telephone a friend or meditate instead, suggests John Foreyt, Ph.D., director of the nutrition research clinic at Baylor College of

long-term success in weight control," says Dr. Callaway. On the other hand, if you don't have the patience to count calories and fat grams, here's an easy rule that will usually point you in the right direction: Focus your eating on whole grains, vegetables, legumes and fruit.

Choose an apple instead of apple juice, brown rice instead of white rice, a whole baked potato instead of french fries, or a fresh apricot instead of an apricot Danish. The less-processed versions are likely to contain less sugar, less fat and more nutrients. And most important for weight watchers, they tend to contain more fiber, which fills you up, so you feel more satisfied on fewer calories. Fiber minimizes insulin response, so less fat is stored.

Medicine in Houston. Most cravings will pass in ten minutes.

BUY INDIVIDUALLY WRAPPED PORTIONS. "It's better to buy a box of fudge pops than a half-gallon of ice cream," says Kostas. "You have built-in portion control."

LISTEN TO YOUR MOUTH. Maybe it's a particular texture you crave. "When my clients crave potato chips, I often refer them to pretzels, popcorn or dry cereals that supply the same crunch," says Kostas.

GO FOR CONTROLLED INDULGENCE. Many of today's fat-free cookies and cakes substitute nicely in a pinch. Just beware of the high caloric toll that some take and limit your intake accordingly. When nothing but the worst will do? "Don't deny yourself," says Dr. Callaway; just set limits. Savoring one decadently rich chocolate truffle can be quite satisfying. Denial sets us up for bingeing and undermines our long-term success.

Part III

Healing with Vitamins: The Year's Breakthroughs

Vitamins and Beyond

Choosing the Ultimate Multivitamin— And More

Diet surveys by the National Institutes of Health (NIH) in Bethesda, Maryland, and the U.S. Department of Agriculture suggest that many Americans routinely get less— often much less—than 100 percent of the Daily Value (DV) for key vitamins and minerals. Even careful eaters may be falling short! When dietitians at Utah State University in Logan tried to design balanced menus that met current dietary guidelines, they had trouble achieving all vitamin and mineral goals for adult women at less than 2,200 calories. That means anyone who usually consumes under 2,200 calories—which includes most women, many dieters and seniors—may fall below at least some DVs. Certain medications also can make you come up short. And slowly and silently, these shortfalls may undermine long-term health.

It's true that experts estimate that for most people, getting only 70 percent of the DVs may be sufficient. That's because DV levels are designed to cover even individuals whose needs are unusually high. But for those people who do have high needs—and there's no practical way yet to identify who they are—getting only 70 percent of the DVs could mean one or more chronic nutrient shortfalls.

Hundreds of studies have linked diets high in essential nutrients to lower rates of disease, though only controlled tests of supplements versus placebos can prove it's the vitamins and minerals that protect us. Nevertheless, some researchers now see chronic illness—such as heart disease, high blood pressure, diabetes and cancer—at least partially as defi-

200

ciency diseases, the way we already think of rickets or scurvy.

The best solution to diet shortfalls? Eating the healthiest foods you can—lots of veggies, fruits, whole grains and low-fat dairy products. Experts suggest it's the potent cocktail of vitamins, minerals, fiber and substances available only in foods that best explains the protective power of healthy diets.

Many experts agree that closing some nutritional gaps with a balanced multiple vitamin/mineral supplement either can't hurt—or just plain makes sense. "It's not a magic bullet, but it is a small, logical insurance policy," says Harvard University epidemiologist Walter Willett, M.D., "especially since there's no evidence of harm." Even many dietitians now take a multi, surveys show.

No research has linked multis to a longer lifespan. But preliminary evidence suggests that multis may increase our "health span," the years that we're free from chronic illness. In a study among people over age 65, use of moderate multis cut the number of days of infection-related illness in half.

The Multis with the Mostest

There's a multitude of multis out there, but many are incomplete (with important nutrients missing or too low) or too complete (with higher-than-warranted doses). So check labels. Your multi should include the following.

Note: Certain supplements can keep you from absorbing prescription medications. (Calcium, for example, can block tetracycline if you take both at the same time.) Ask your pharmacist about potential interactions between supplements and medications.

Vitamin A/beta-carotene. Aim for 100 percent of the DV for vitamin A (5,000 international units), some of which may come from beta-carotene, a vitamin A precursor. (Although there is no DV for beta-carotene, the beta-carotene equivalent of the DV for vitamin A is 3 milligrams.) Diets rich in beta-carotene (an important antioxidant) have been linked to lower rates of lung, breast and many other cancers, heart disease, stroke and cataracts. But whether beta-carotene supplements that supply vitamin A levels well above DV range will be beneficial is controversial and awaiting results of ongoing studies. On the plus side, preliminary results from Harvard's famous Physicians' Health Study show that doctors with heart disease who took 50 milligrams of beta-carotene every other day for six years had half as many strokes, fatal heart attacks and angioplasties as doctors who took placebos.

Beta-carotene supplements also have been associated with regression of oral cancer and lower rates of cancer of the esophagus.

But one surprising study in Finland found that smokers taking 20 milligrams of beta-carotene daily had increased rates of lung cancer. Until we know more, if you choose to add a beta-carotene supplement, a sensible amount is 6 milligrams. (Preformed vitamin A—but not beta-carotene—can be toxic at 50,000 international units.)

Niacin. Your goal should be to get 100 percent of the DV (20 milligrams). Niacin at high doses (more than 1,000 milligrams) is useful for some heart patients because it raises high-density lipoproteins (HDLs), the "good" cholesterol, and lowers triglycerides. But because of the possibility of serious side effects, including liver damage—especially from slow-release niacin—these super-high doses must be taken only under a doctor's supervision.

Folic acid. Try to get 100 percent of the DV, listed on labels either as 400 micrograms or 0.4 milligrams. Surveys show that many Americans, and most women, are falling far short of these levels. Getting enough of this emerging superstar vitamin is the number one reason to take a multi supplement, says Meir Stampfer, M.D., professor of epidemiology and nutrition at the Harvard School of Public Health. The U.S. Public Health Service urges all women of childbearing age to get 400 micrograms of folic acid daily to help prevent babies born with serious brain and spinal cord defects.

Beyond this, diets low in folic acid are linked to high blood levels of homocysteine, a newly studied substance strongly linked to heart disease. Diets high in folic acid appear to be linked to lower risks of cervical and colon cancer.

Vitamin B₆. Aim for 100 percent of the DV (2 milligrams). As with folic acid, American diets are low in B₆ (and for some women, long-term use of oral contraceptives appears to increase B₆ needs). Low B₆ intakes are linked to high homocysteine levels and greater heart attack risk and poor functioning of the immune system in older people. The reported benefits of high levels of B₆ supplements for carpal tunnel syndrome or premenstrual syndrome are not yet confirmed. Caution: Megadoses of 500 milligrams per day (250 times the DV) have been associated with nerve damage. And problems have been associated with B₆ at intakes as low as 50 milligrams.

Vitamin B₁₂. Shoot for 100 percent of the DV (6 micrograms). Here's yet another B vitamin linked to higher levels of homocysteine and heart disease in those who consume or absorb the least. Lack of enough B₁₂ in the elderly is also associated with memory loss and disorientation, symptoms that can mimic Alzheimer's disease. Since older people may have trouble absorbing B₁₂, any suspected deficiencies in this age group should be treated by a physician. Total vegetarians may especially need to supplement, because B₁₂ is found almost exclusively in animal products.

Vitamin D. You should try to get 100 percent of the DV (400 international units). You need enough vitamin D to make it possible to absorb the calcium you eat (though you don't have to consume the two nutrients at the same time). Good sources are sunshine on the skin and vitamin D–fortified milk. For those who can't achieve adequate vitamin D intake through diet, supplements may be the simplest solution, according to Bess Dawson-Hughes, M.D., chief of the calcium and bone metabolism lab at the Jean Mayer USDA Human Nutrition Research Center on Aging in Boston. Don't supplement more than 400 international units without your doctor's supervision; high levels can be toxic.

Copper. Shoot for 100 percent of the DV (2 milligrams). Copper acts as part of an important antioxidant enzyme system that seems to play a role in heart health. According to USDA vitamin and mineral specialist Richard Anderson,

Ph.D., however, most Americans' diets supply less than half the copper they need. Above all, make sure any multi that has 100 percent of the DV for zinc (15 milligrams) also has 100 percent of the DV for copper—some don't. Elevating zinc intake without taking in enough copper can lead to copper deficiency, Dr. Anderson cautions.

Iron. Premenopausal women should aim for 100 percent of the DV (18 milligrams). Men and postmenopausal women should aim for 0 to 50 percent of the DV (0 to 9 milligrams). Women having periods—especially those with heavy bleeding—or women who exercise may well need a supplement to ensure they get enough iron, though they should not take more than 18 milligrams unless diagnosed with iron deficiency anemia. In that case, iron supplementation should be directed by your physician. In men and postmenopausal women, levels of body iron stores rise with age.

High levels of iron have been associated with increased risk of heart attack in some studies, though other studies find no link. Until we know more, some experts think it's sensible to choose a supplement light in iron if you're a postmenopausal woman or a man.

Magnesium. Your goal should be to get 100 milligrams of magnesium a day, which is 25 percent of the DV (400 milligrams), the most you're likely to find in a single-dose supplement. (Otherwise, the capsule would be too big to swallow.) Diets low in magnesium have been linked to high blood pressure, and the NIH now recommends adequate magnesium intake as one part of a lifestyle to avoid high blood pressure. Small studies have shown that magnesium supplements can help reduce elevated blood pressure and may improve insulin sensitivity in some people who have diabetes.

Though diet surveys show that most Americans' diets are low in magnesium, an extra 100 milligrams in your multi may be enough to put you in pretty good shape, says Judith Hallfrisch, Ph.D., research leader of the metabolism and nutrient interactions laboratory at the USDA Human Nutrition Research Center in Beltsville, Maryland. Or to be certain, you might want to consider adding magnesium as a single supplement at no more than 400 milligrams.

Excess magnesium can lead to diarrhea. Those with abnormal kidney function should not supplement magnesium without a doctor's supervision.

Zinc. Aim for 100 percent of the DV (15 milligrams). Zinc is known to be necessary for proper wound healing and a strong immune system. Yet surveys by Dr. Hallfrisch and others show that it may be the mineral most lacking in U.S. diets. Zinc supplements improved signs of immune function in two studies among elderly people at risk for zinc deficiency at Wayne State University in Detroit and in France. (Paradoxically, supplementing with too much zinc—25 milligrams a day in one study—may backfire and weaken the immune system.)

Chromium. Aim for 50 to 200 micrograms, a safe range set by the National Research Council. Supplements may be

Does Your Multi Pack Enough Calcium?

"Complete! Total! Balanced!" No matter what the label lingo shouts (or only hints), don't assume that a women's formula supplies the right amount of every vitamin or mineral a woman needs. In fact, some multiples have only a fraction of the one nutrient women probably need most—calcium.

The truth is, no single-dose multi tablet or capsule can possibly contain 100 percent of the Daily Value (DV) for calcium—the pill would have to be bigger than a super-colossal olive!

Also, some women's formulas contain too much iron—as much as 40 milligrams. No woman should take more than 100 percent of the DV (18 milligrams) unless her doctor so advises. And after menopause, women should consider taking less than 100 percent.

The moral is, check to see if your women's formula is a good multi, then fill in the missing calcium.

the only way for most of us to get enough chromium: Studies by Dr. Anderson demonstrate that it's difficult to get even the minimum 50 micrograms of chromium on less than 3,000 calories a day. Chromium forms part of a substance called glucose-tolerance factor that helps our cells absorb the blood sugar we convert to energy. Very preliminary research indicates that chromium supplements may improve glucose handling in people with diabetes and shrink elevated cholesterol levels. Research showing that chromium may promote weight loss and develop muscle mass is conflicting at this time.

Selenium. Aim for 70 to 100 micrograms, a safe range suggested by our experts. Selenium plays a role in a powerful antioxidant enzyme, glutathione peroxidase. In China, selenium supplements (combined with supplements of beta-carotene and vitamin E) reduced the risk of dying from cancer among a large population deficient in these nutrients. In Italy, deaths from heart disease rose dramatically among residents of a village whose public water supply was changed from wells high in selenium to water with a lower selenium content. Stay in the recommended safe range; selenium is toxic at higher intakes, particularly over 1 milligram per day.

Moving Beyond a Multi

Prevention magazine thinks there's good reason to add three more single supplements to your program. They are calcium, vitamin C and vitamin E.

Calcium. If you're a woman, chances are strong that you need a separate calcium supplement, because no single-dose multi that we've seen contains 100 percent of the DV—1,000 milligrams. (Most multis have 200 milligrams or less.) It's clear from many studies that adequate calcium lowers risks of osteoporosis, the bone-thinning disease that affects half of all women over age 50. Yet, according to Dr. Hallfrisch, "It's very difficult for women to get all the calcium they need from diet alone—unless they're crazy about milk." (Adequate calcium intake may also help prevent high blood pressure and preeclampsia, some research shows.)

Your goal: All women ages 25 to 50 and men ages 25 to 65: 1,000 milligrams. Young adults under 25: 1,200 to 1,500 milligrams.

All women over 50 and men over 65: 1,500 milligrams, or 150 percent of the DV. (These are NIH recommendations.) To determine how much calcium you need to supplement, find your goal. Then subtract 300 milligrams for each serving of milk, yogurt, cheese or calcium-fortified orange juice you normally consume as well as the amount of calcium in your multi. Many women need 500 to 1,000 milligrams of supplemental calcium a day.

Your Supplement Checklist

Are all supplements alike? Not quite. Here's what to look for—in multis and in single supplements.

Multiple vitamin/mineral supplement: Make sure your formula provides all of the following:

- 100 percent of the DV for vitamin A/beta-carotene, niacin, vitamin B_6, vitamin B_{12}, folic acid, vitamin D, copper and zinc. Other nutrients also may be present at up to 100 percent of DV levels.
- Chromium: 50 to 200 micrograms
- Selenium: 70 to 100 micrograms
- Iron: Men and postmenopausal women: 0 to 50 percent of the DV (0 to 9 milligrams). Premenopausal women: 100 percent of the DV.
- Magnesium: 25 percent of the DV (100 milligrams). Accept no less in a single-dose multi.

Calcium supplement: 500 to 1,000 milligrams. Usually this requires more than one tablet.

Vitamin C supplement: 100 to 500 milligrams.

Vitamin E supplement: 100 to 400 international units.

Citrate vs. carbonate: Before age 60 people seem to absorb all forms of calcium equally well. After 60, try to take calcium carbonate with meals to ensure absorption. Most older people can absorb calcium citrate on an empty stomach.

Lead levels: Avoid supplements made from bone meal, dolomite and oyster shell ("natural source" calcium carbonate); they may contain too much lead.

Chewables: These are useful if you have trouble swallowing calcium tablets. And flavored varieties are now available. Or look for a citrus-flavored drinkable calcium supplement—you make it from tablets that dissolve in water.

Elemental calcium: It's the milligrams of "elemental" cal-

Multis: A User's Glossary

Is reading the label of your multivitamin supplement like trying to read a foreign language? Here's a guide to understanding what's in your multi and how best to take it.

Expiration date. A reputable supplement will carry one, though you may need a pharmacist's help to find it. For optimum potency, don't buy supplements that you can't use up before that time.

Ability to dissolve. Look for multis to start displaying the letters "USP," a promise to dissolve 75 percent after one hour in body fluids, according to recently changed standards of the (nongovernmental) U.S. Pharmacopeia.

Bioavailability. Look for iron as ferrous sulfate or ferrous fumarate, the most absorbable forms. Experts say the chemical form of other nutrients in multis doesn't make a significant difference.

Natural versus synthetic. Experts agree there's no important difference.

Timed-release multis. They're supposed to sustain steady blood levels of nutrients. But they may

cium in your supplement that count. If the label doesn't reveal this, just add a zero to the percent DV. For example, a label says that four tablets provide 50 percent of the DV. That means four tablets provide 500 milligrams of elemental calcium.

Disintegration: Experts agree this is no longer a problem with major national and store brands.

Divide your dose: Best absorption occurs with doses of 500 milligrams or less at a time.

Bedtime snack: Taking a calcium supplement at bedtime may protect bones by keeping parathyroid hormone levels from rising during the night. Parathyroid hormone causes bone to lose calcium.

---

release nutrients in the gastrointestinal tract past the point where they're absorbed.

Divided-dose multis. These are multis that are sold in divided doses that you take several times during the day. If you're very motivated, these multis are your best bet to keep blood levels of nutrients steady all day.

When to take supplements. For maximum absorption, take your multi with meals, not on an empty stomach. And make sure the meal isn't totally fat-free: Fat-soluble vitamins in multis such as beta-carotene/vitamin A, vitamin D and vitamin E need three to five grams of fat—equal to about a teaspoon of margarine—to get inside you.

Storage. To preserve the potency of multis, avoid storing them in hot or humid places such as the bathroom, a sunny windowsill, over the sink or by the stove. Don't keep them in the refrigerator, either. Many experts suggest using the cupboard where you keep spices.

Wheat bran: Avoid taking supplements along with high-fiber wheat bran cereals (10 grams or more of fiber). They can reduce calcium absorption by 25 percent.

Constipation: Some people report constipation with calcium carbonate. Try calcium citrate if this is a problem.

Safety: Don't take supplements of calcium totaling above 2,000 milligrams a day unless your doctor prescribes it. If you have kidney stones, check with your doctor, though recent research indicates that calcium does not increase kidney stone formation.

Vitamin C. There's evidence that intake of this antioxidant vitamin at levels above the DV (60 milligrams) may have added protective effects. During a large ten-year government study, men consuming an average of 300 milligrams of vitamin C per day (partly from supplements) had almost half the deaths from heart disease of men taking in less than 50 milligrams a day. Preliminary research shows that higher vitamin C intake is associated with higher HDL and lower total and low-density lipoprotein, or LDL, cholesterol levels.

Intake of high vitamin C foods has been linked to protection against cancers of the digestive tract, cervix, rectum, breast and lung (though studies using C supplements are inconclusive). And even if you don't smoke, your blood levels of vitamin C can be depleted by breathing secondhand smoke, a study conducted at the University of California at Berkeley showed.

Your goal: 100 to 500 milligrams.

Natural vs. synthetic: Experts say there's no significant difference.

Pass up chewable C: Large, regular doses (500 milligrams or more) of chewable C can raise levels of acid in the mouth and threaten tooth enamel. Stick to C you can swallow.

Safety: Vitamin C at 100 to 500 milligrams appears to be safe—you'd get 100 milligrams of vitamin C in an eight-ounce glass of orange juice from concentrate, for example. *Note:* Diarrhea sometimes occurs at intakes of 1,000 milligrams or more.

Vitamin E. Here's another key antioxidant vitamin that *Prevention* magazine thinks makes sense to take at levels above the DV (30 international units). Two large observational studies among nurses and male health professionals found that those taking at least 100 IU of vitamin E (as supplements) for at least two years had a risk of heart disease approximately 40 percent lower than those who consumed about 10 international units a day through diet alone.

Higher levels of vitamin E appear to boost signs of immune function in the elderly, according to recent research. Preliminary evidence suggests that supplements or high intakes of vitamin E may reduce risks of cataracts and some cancers and may have some positive effects for people with diabetes.

But to get vitamin E at levels that appear to be protective, you must supplement. You'd need to consume more than 2 cups of corn oil or approximately 1½ cups of peanut butter, for example, to get 100 international units!

Your goal: 100 to 400 international units.

Natural vs. synthetic: 100 international units of synthetic E is equal in potency to 100 international units of natural E. Although the much more expensive natural E is more active inside the body than synthetic E, the international unit is a unit designed to equalize this difference.

Take E with some fat: Vitamin E needs fat to get absorbed. Most E capsules include a minute amount of oil (about 0.02 grams of fat). That's not enough, experts believe, to maximize absorption. You probably need 3 to 5 grams of fat (equal to one teaspoon of margarine), an amount present in most meals, as long as they're not fat-free.

Safety: Vitamin E at 100 to 400 international units appears to be safe for almost everyone. But because a recent study in Finland showed a slightly increased risk of stroke due to hemorrhage, if you're on blood-thinning medicine, you should check with your doctor.

Antioxidants

Added Protection against Arthritis and Cancer

STEAM SOME BROCCOLI. Toss it in rosemary-infused olive oil. That tasty side dish may also be Teflon for your joints. That's because it contains vitamin E, beta-carotene and selenium, a trio of nutrients that scientists hope can save you from ever feeling the ache of rheumatoid arthritis.

Deactivating Arthritis

Some research has hinted that antioxidant vitamins like these may thwart some of the joint damage once you have the disease. But a recent study from Finland looked at whether they'd help you stave off the disease in the first place. Researchers looked at blood samples from 1,419 volunteers, then watched who developed arthritis over 20 years. They found that people with the lowest levels of vitamin E, beta-carotene and selenium in their blood were eight times more likely than people with the highest levels to develop that disease.

It's suspected that arthritis has many different origins. "It's possible that the diet is a contributing factor," says David S. Pisetsky, M.D., Ph.D., medical adviser to the Arthritis Foundation and author of *The Duke University Medical Center Book of Arthritis*.

It's known that when the disease is in full swing, free radicals (harmful, unstable molecules that antioxidant vitamins may help muzzle) can damage the joints. But the question of how—and if—the vitamins might hold off the ache in the first place is still murky.

More studies need to be done to determine whether anti-oxidants could be a glimmer of hope for prevention. For now, foods high in these antioxidants are a pretty sensible strategy no matter what your motivation. You've probably already found your favorite sources of vitamin E and beta-carotene. And as a refresher, selenium is found in canned tuna and salmon, and it's also found in smaller amounts in broccoli, celery, cucumbers, mushrooms and grains.

Squelching Cancer Comebacks

You give bladder cancer the surgical oust, only to have it play the Elvis trick of reappearing—usually more than once. Immunization, a standard bladder cancer therapy, has been somewhat effective in blocking this boomerang effect that occurs in nearly 88 percent of bladder cancer cases. But one study hints that megadoses of vitamins may do much more to block it.

Researchers pitted the Daily Value (DV) of vitamins A, B_6, C and E and zinc against megadoses of these nutrients. (Dosages were, respectively, 8, 50, 33, 13 and 6 times the DV. So don't even think of trying this yourself.) All 65 people, who already had a go-round with the disease, also received immunization therapy. After four years the megadose group had a 40 percent decrease in the recurrence of tumors over the DV group.

"One possible explanation for the results is that the vita-min treatment may be stimulating the immune system to fight off the cancer," says study leader Donald L. Lamm, M.D., chair of the Department of Urology at West Virginia University in Morgantown. It's not yet clear whether one vitamin is outdoing the rest, he says, "and it's possible that the combination is better than any single ingredient." That combination may be powerful enough to fight a good battle against cancer recurrence even without the help of immunization therapy, he speculates, though with this small study, it's hard to tell absolutely.

Questions remain about the safety of megadoses, and

additional studies may tweak the balance of vitamins. But this study offers new hope against bladder cancer's seemingly endless sequels.

The Mighty Bs
Can These Vitamins Disarm a Heart-Harming Villain?

HOMOCYSTEINE IS A SUBSTANCE you've probably never heard of. But rest assured you'll be hearing plenty in the next few years. The fact is, in persons with very elevated blood levels of homocysteine (a condition called hyperhomocysteinemia), the risk of premature vascular disease is 30 times greater than it is for those with normal levels. And even in people who don't have this condition, higher levels of homocysteine have been linked to greater heart disease risk.

On the other hand, if high levels of homocysteine are a threat to heart health, there may be a simple way to lower these levels: B vitamins. In particular, three B vitamins—B_6, B_{12} and folic acid—seem to work.

Unmasking Homocysteine

A pair of high-profile studies in recent years have uncovered the surprising facts about homocysteine. In the Physicians' Health Study (the study that yielded the news that aspirin prevents heart attacks), researchers compared homocysteine levels of the 5 percent of people having the highest levels of homocysteine with most of the other people who had lower levels. Those in the top 5 percent (highest levels) were linked to a dramatic 3.4-fold greater risk of heart attack.

To get an idea of the significance of this 3.4-fold elevation in risk, compare that number with the dangers from elevated cholesterol: If you started with a healthy 180 cholesterol level, you'd have to get all the way up to 270 to see a comparable jump in risk.

According to Meir Stampfer, M.D., professor of epidemiology and nutrition at the Harvard School of Public Health, who led the Physicians' Health Study, the data seemed to indicate that only those with the highest levels of homocysteine were at increased cardiovascular risk.

"Obviously, for people with a high level of homocysteine, it's important to bring that level down. But even at average levels, it may turn out to be a worthwhile idea to lower levels further," says Dr. Stampfer.

Now it could be that homocysteine is just a marker for some other physiological factor that's the real cause of greater heart disease risk. After all, this study shows only that there's some kind of association between homocysteine and heart disease. But if homocysteine itself is a true culprit, the hope is that consuming the three B vitamins mentioned above will lower your risk of cardiovascular disease. And there's some reason for optimism.

Following the Physicians' Health Study, data from the long-running Framingham Heart Study showed that the lower the blood levels of the three Bs, the higher the blood levels of homocysteine. And here's the big shocker: People in the study didn't have to be vitamin-deficient before homocysteine levels rose. Even nutrient levels above the current Daily Values (DVs) were linked to higher homocysteine levels.

Taking a Closer Look

Researchers first started examining homocysteine levels three decades ago when it was discovered that children with a genetic disorder leading to premature cardiovascular disease had very elevated levels of the substance. Ironically, the extreme levels of homocysteine found in these persons drew attention away from the possibility that people with relatively slight elevations (compared with those with the genetic disorder) could also be at risk.

"We used to think it was only those with a rare genetic disease, homocystinuria, who were at risk for heart disease," says James Finkelstein, M.D., a pioneer researcher in the field who is chief of medical service at the Veterans' Administration

Good Sources of Heart-Healthy B Vitamins

Want to start to treat your heart to more Bs? Here's what you should be munching.

FOOD	VITAMIN CONTENT
VITAMIN B$_6$ (mg.)	
DAILY VALUE: 2 mg.	
I medium baked potato	0.91
I medium banana	0.73
I serving (as shown on label) B$_6$-fortified cereal	0.50
3 ounces broiled beef, top round	0.48
3 ounces baked halibut	0.34
3 ounces baked swordfish	0.32
I cup cooked brown rice	0.28
½ cup cooked spinach	0.22
½ cup cooked peas	0.17
½ cup cooked navy beans	0.15
½ avocado	0.14
½ cup cooked chick-peas	0.11
VITAMIN B$_{12}$ (mcg.)	
DAILY VALUE: 6 mcg.	
3 ounces baked Atlantic mackerel	16.0
I cup New England clam chowder	10.0
3 ounces braised beef, lean chuck	2.9

Medical Center and professor of medicine at George Washington and Howard Universities, all in Washington, D.C. "We now know differently. Persons who are at the high end of the normal range for blood levels of homocysteine can still be at greatly increased risk of arteriosclerosis," he says.

If the idea that hyperhomocysteinemia may be a possible

FOOD	VITAMIN CONTENT
3 ounces canned tuna	1.9
1 serving (as shown on label) B$_{12}$-fortified cereal	1.5
1 cup skim milk	0.9
½ cup tempeh	0.8
½ cup 1% low-fat cottage cheese	0.7

FOLIC ACID (mg.)

DAILY VALUE: 0.4 mg.

½ cup cooked baby lima beans	0.14
½ cup cooked chick-peas	0.14
½ cup cooked spinach	0.13
½ cup cooked red kidney beans	0.11
1 cup orange juice, from frozen concentrate	0.11
1 serving (as shown on label) folic acid- or folate-fortified cereal	0.10
4 spears cooked asparagus	0.06
½ cup cooked beets	0.05
1 medium orange	0.05
½ cup cooked broccoli	0.04

risk factor becomes more widespread, testing for homocysteine levels may become routine, speculates Jacob Selhub, Ph.D., of the Jean Mayer USDA Human Nutrition Research Center on Aging at Tufts University in Boston and a principal investigator of the study on homocysteine and B vitamins in the Framingham population. Right now, testing would be prohibitively expensive in most cases.

Another kink in the story is that homocysteine is formed from a protein component (amino acid) called methionine. Methionine is found in all proteins but shows particularly high levels in meat.

This raises an interesting question: Could you lower homocysteine levels by consuming less of the methionine it is made from? That is, by consuming less meat? "Probably," says Dr. Finkelstein. "Methionine is essential to the body, which uses it to form proteins and take part in a variety of reactions. But beyond a certain level, you don't need any more methionine in the diet. Above this level you could probably bring homocysteine down by reducing methionine intake."

Nevertheless, homocysteine isn't by itself a bad thing. Homocysteine takes part in a variety of important biochemical reactions, including conversion to methionine, formation of cysteine (a second amino acid with many important functions) and others.

Here's where the three Bs come into play: Each one—folic acid, B_6 and B_{12}—plays a role in converting homocysteine into nontoxic compounds. When your body is deficient in one of the three Bs, it cannot efficiently alter homocysteine. And because these enzymes often work in tandem, you may need all three Bs to drive homocysteine to its lowest level.

Take Prudent Action Now

Researchers agree that B vitamins are not a magic bullet against homocysteine or, for that matter, heart disease. "For one thing, B vitamins will ordinarily do nothing to correct a genetic enzyme deficiency," explains Rowena Matthews, Ph.D., professor of biological chemistry at the University of

Michigan Biophysics Research Division in Ann Arbor.

Then there's the matter of whether the three Bs—which we strongly suspect lower homocysteine—will actually prove, in turn, to lower heart attack risk. "We expect it will," says Dr. Selhub. "But we don't know that. Clinical trials must be conducted."

Researchers agree, though, that until more is known about the relationship among homocysteine, B vitamins and heart disease, your best bet seems to be to make sure you're getting enough Bs in your diet. "With lowering blood pressure and cholesterol, people are forever hearing what they shouldn't eat," says Dr. Selhub. "But when it comes to lowering homocysteine, we get to tell people all the foods they should eat for heart health."

Indeed, the news is deliciously healthy: Folic acid (also known as folate) can be found in orange juice, greens, such as broccoli and spinach, and legumes, including navy, lima and kidney beans. Rich sources of B_6 include bananas, baked potatoes (with the skin), peas and avocados. Besides these natural sources, many cereals are fortified with 25 percent of the DV for both folic acid and vitamin B_6 per serving. (Check the labels to find ones that are high in these vitamins.)

Vitamin B_{12}, however, poses a nutritional dilemma. Some of the best B_{12} sources are also high in saturated fat and cholesterol (beef liver and lamb kidney, for example). But that doesn't mean you can't get plenty of this vitamin with some careful menu planning. For example, a three-ounce slice of lean beef, a bowl of B_{12}-fortified cereal and an eight-ounce cup of skim milk provide nearly all the DV of B_{12}.

It's true that since the vitamin is present in significant amounts only in animal foods, strict vegetarians—those who do not eat meat, eggs or dairy foods—can come up short and may need to take care to include fermented soy products in their diets (such as tempeh), which are rich in B_{12}, or take B_{12} supplements. In addition, elderly vegetarians and nonvegetarians alike are at increased risk for B_{12} deficiency, explains Robert H. Allen, M.D., professor of medicine and head of the Division of Hematology at the University of Colorado Health

Sciences Center in Denver. B_{12} relies primarily on three compounds that work together to effectively release it into the body: hydrochloric acid, the enzyme pepsin and a protein called intrinsic factor. As the years go by, however, our bodies produce less of these compounds, so B_{12} absorption may be severely impaired. In fact, by the time a person reaches age 70, there is a 50 percent chance that he will have a marked decrease in hydrochloric acid and pepsin production. As a result, older people may need oral supplements (check with your doctor first) or require injections of B_{12}. For those who are concerned that they may not be getting enough B vitamins in their diets, Dr. Stampfer recommends a multivitamin supplement providing the DV of B_6, B_{12}, folic acid and other vital nutrients.

The DV for vitamin B_6 is 2 milligrams; for B_{12}, 6 micrograms and for folic acid, 0.4 milligrams. Supplements of these Bs should not widely exceed these recommendations because of the risk of side effects.

The findings on homocysteine and heart disease may go a long way toward explaining heart disease where none of the standard risk factors—smoking, high blood pressure or elevated cholesterol—are present. And the findings on the three Bs show us there's more reason than ever to focus on good nutrition.

....

Vitamin C
Can It Stem Complications from Diabetes?

PEOPLE WITH DIABETES may have already heard about ongoing research to see if vitamin C can reduce the risk of heart disease. Now a study has hinted that the vitamin may stop the body from producing sorbitol, a compound made from glucose that may be an instigator in kidney, retina and nerve damage. Don't let the name of the compound confuse you: The sorbitol used as a sweetener takes a different route and doesn't cause damage like the sorbitol made in your cells.

Researchers gave vitamin C doses of either 100 milligrams (about what's in eight ounces, or one cup, of orange juice) or 600 milligrams to 9 people with diabetes and 11 people without. Within 30 days of this two-month study, people with diabetes who had more than average sorbitol at the start saw levels come under control. The higher-dose vitamin had greater—but not dramatically different—effects. Sorbitol levels in individuals without diabetes remained essentially the same as when they began.

It's a bit of a mystery how vitamin C could come to the aid of these vulnerable organs. Nonetheless, "if vitamin C in these doses proves to inhibit the production of sorbitol, this could be exciting," says Kathleen Wishner, M.D., Ph.D. president of the American Diabetes Association and associate clinical professor of medicine at the University of Southern California, Los Angeles. "The problem with the other drugs that have been proposed to do this is that they've all had side effects. As far as we know, there are no side effects to these doses of vitamin C."

Even if future studies confirm that vitamin C does inhibit the buildup of sorbitol, researchers may find that sorbitol has more than one accomplice in creating these complications with diabetes. Dr. Wishner suggests that an extra 100 milligrams of doctor-sanctioned vitamin C (found not just in eight ounces of orange juice but also in 1½ cups of cantaloupe or a red pepper) may not harm people with diabetes. But the best way to give complications a wide berth is to keep tight control over diabetes.

Vitamin E

A New Ally
in Stroke Treatment

ALL THAT GOOD EATING and aspirin-taking may add up to more if you've had a ministroke and your doctor tells you to take vitamin E. Recent research suggests that this vitamin may be a sidekick that helps aspirin fend off strokes in susceptible people.

Researchers warded off strokes with the standard strategy—aspirin—in 48 people who had small, warning-type strokes called transient ischemic attacks (TIAs). Fifty-two other people who had TIAs added 400 international units of vitamin E to their aspirin routines. (The Daily Value, or DV, for vitamin E is only 30 international units, so don't try this at home.) After two years people taking the dynamic vitamin/aspirin duo had a 25 percent reduced risk of a potentially damaging stroke compared with those who took aspirin alone. Compare that with what would happen if you did nothing, and you find that the combination may offer a 45 percent reduction in stroke risk.

The theory is that the double-pill regimen does more than one thing to stop stroke. Vitamin E may reduce the chance that an injured vessel wall will look like an appealing home to platelets. (Platelets assist in the clotting of blood.) Aspirin may help stop platelets from forming a gang among themselves. Either way, chances get smaller that clumped blood factors will break off and cork up arteries downstream.

Study leader Manfred Steiner, M.D., Ph.D., professor of medicine, hematology/oncology section, at East Carolina University School of Medicine in Greenville, North Carolina, says that the key is to talk with your doctor before you do anything, since these anticlotting strategies can work *too* well and cause bleeding.

But if future studies confirm these benefits, says Dr. Steiner, "I think the use of vitamin E with aspirin could become standard."

....

Folate
Cereal Offers Stroke Protection

MAYBE YOU DON'T GET the decoder ring. But inside some of those adult cereals you've been eating might be Captain Mystic himself. Cereals that are fortified with folate (as well as other foods that contain this nutrient) may have the power to spare you from stroke, according to recent research.

Sometimes it's called folic acid, and sometimes it's called folacin. Either way, this nutrient holds back blood levels of a chemical called homocysteine. Experts believe that too much homocysteine may predispose you to heart disease. (See "The Mighty Bs" on page 214.) A recent study suggests it may be a bad actor in stroke, too.

Researchers checked the homocysteine levels of 109 men who developed strokes against the levels of 427 men who didn't. They found that the highest levels were associated with a slightly elevated risk of stroke. Current thinking suggests that homocysteine plays a role in injury to vessel walls, in changes of the low-density lipoprotein, or LDL, cholesterol on those walls, or in clot formation—all of which can lead to stroke.

Researchers used to believe that vitamins B_6, B_{12} and folate all had roles in reining in runaway homocysteine. But when 100 men with high homocysteine levels in South Africa were given either 650 micrograms of folate, 0.4 milligrams of vitamin B_{12}, 10 milligrams of B_6 or a combination of all three vitamins for six weeks, researchers found that the combination of vitamins cut homocysteine levels almost in half. But folate alone did nearly the same thing.

"Folate is the key player," says Meir Stampfer, M.D., professor of epidemiology and nutrition at the Harvard School of Public Health. "This study showed that clearer and nicer than ever before." The nutrient is believed to hurry the metabolism of homocysteine into a more benign substance.

In the future homocysteine tests could be as routine as cholesterol tests. But for now, those prohibitively expensive tests are only done at major medical centers. There's no way to guess at your level without doing the test, except to know that low levels of folate have been linked to (and are suspected to be a cause of) high homocysteine levels.

The Daily Value for folate is 400 micrograms. Four hundred micrograms would look like this: one cup of orange juice (110 micrograms), one cup of folate-fortified cereal (160 micrograms) plus a cup of raw spinach with lunch or dinner (130 micrograms). Other good sources include lima beans, chick-peas, kidney and navy beans, wheat germ and broccoli.

But if you are depending on your breakfast cereal to give you a head start on this nutrient, read the label. Folate can fool you: Some cereals with plenty of good stuff have eleven times less folate than even cereals that seem more like dessert.

....

Lecithin

A Nutrient to Jog Your Memory

THE POWER OF LECITHIN as a booster for memory is intriguing but unproven. Human research with lecithin or its component, choline—primarily among Alzheimer's patients—

has been conflicting. But there's a promising study that *Prevention* magazine would like to see confirmed in follow-up research.

Forty-one healthy people ages 50 to 80 took two tablespoons of lecithin granules a day (13.5 grams lecithin, which provided 500 milligrams of choline). After five weeks these folks had reduced memory lapses—episodes of forgetting names, having a word on the tips of their tongues or misplacing things. The lapses decreased from an average 35 a week to 19 a week compared with those people who took a placebo. Researcher Florence Safford, doctor of social work and associate professor in the School of Social Work at Florida International University in North Miami, reported that one woman realized that her memory must have been improving when she noticed her refrigerator door sported only half the number of yellow stick-it reminders she normally posted.

Though the body makes its own choline, some experts such as Steven Zeisel, M.D., Ph.D., chairman of the nutrition department at the University of North Carolina at Chapel Hill, believe we may not make enough, so we need choline from our diets, too. (Since choline is widely found in food, an absolute deficiency is probably rare.) But the top food sources of choline—high-lecithin foods such as liver, egg yolks and peanuts—are also high in dietary cholesterol and fat, culprits we're cutting back on to protect our hearts. Since two Food and Drug Administration reports have concluded that lecithin supplements in the 13.5-gram range are safe, Dr. Zeisel and Dr. Safford both agree that it would be reasonable for people troubled by memory loss to try lecithin supplements under the guidance of a physician. There's no guarantee the supplements will help, however.

Lecithin granules can be sprinkled on cereal (they dissolve in milk) or mixed with juice.

Note: Each tablespoon of lecithin granules contains 60 calories and about 5.5 grams of fat. Lecithin is *not* recommended at higher doses for anyone with a history of depression or who has trouble digesting fat.

···

Magnesium

Can This Mineral Knock Back Asthma?

ARE TRIPS TO THE SALAD BAR an asthma deterrent? Maybe. Recent research suggests that eating magnesium-dense foods may help stop asthma in its tracks.

It's known that magnesium plays a role in helping relax the muscles lining our breathing passages. A recent study suggests that a low-magnesium diet may up the risk of asthma, a disease characterized by constrictions of those passages. Researchers in England tested over 2,500 adults, exposing them to a chemical that triggers constricted airways in asthma patients. They found that those people with the lowest-magnesium diets were twice as likely to experience this reaction as people with the highest-magnesium diets.

Most Americans' diets fall well below 400 milligrams, the Daily Value (DV) for magnesium. To maximize intake, lead scientist John Britton, M.D., recommends eating more foods rich in magnesium—whole grains, wheat bran and wheat germ, dark green vegetables, such as spinach and broccoli, beans and nuts. Future research will explore whether magnesium supplements can ease symptoms for asthma patients. So for now, use magnesium supplements above DV levels only under a doctor's supervision.

Potassium and Other Minerals
Eating to Ease High Blood Pressure

YOU'RE NOT GOING TO EAT the potato chips. You refuse. You push them off your plate where the waiter has artfully piled them, dump them onto an extra plate and ask that they be removed from sight.

This isn't some little diet trick du jour, either. You're fighting in favor of your blood pressure. Your father's doctor said that salty foods—foods such as potato chips, nuts and lunchmeats—raised your father's blood pressure and helped set him up for his stroke. So not even one small, salted chipette will find its evil little way into your mouth to cause the same problem. It's simply not going to happen to you.

Trying to lower high blood pressure so you don't end up with a stroke, heart attack or kidney disease—the three major health consequences of high blood pressure—is wonderful. But this particular antisalt strategy may backfire. Because some researchers are now saying that by avoiding salt, you may be creating the very health threat that you're trying to avoid. Instead, high blood pressure is just as likely to be caused by low levels of potassium, magnesium and calcium in your body.

Taking a New Look at Salt

Until a few years ago no one really had a handle on what makes blood pressure rise and fall. That's beginning to change.

"A rise in blood pressure means you need to add minerals to your diet, *not* cut back on salt," says David McCarron, M.D., head of the Division of Nephrology, Hypertension and Clinical Pharmacology and director of the National Institute of Diabetes, Digestive and Kidney Diseases' Clinical Nutrition Research Center at Oregon Health Sciences University in Portland. "Tragically, the idea that salt is bad for your blood pressure is one of the most generally accepted notions out there."

It's constantly repeated because an entire generation of doctors didn't have the research that now clarifies the connection between salt (about 40 percent sodium and 60 percent chloride) and other nutrients. Dr. McCarron explains that in

Food Factors

Although vitamins and minerals clearly play a significant role in preventing and perhaps treating high blood pressure, other dietary strategies can also help keep your blood pressure where it belongs.

CUT CALORIES. Obesity is one of the biggest risk factors for high blood pressure, reports the National Heart, Lung and Blood Institute in Bethesda, Maryland. It can make you two to six times more likely to develop the problem than if you were at a healthier weight. That's why the National Institute suggests that you lose weight by cutting back 500 calories a day—and finding ways to burn off even more by becoming more physically active.

EAT FISH. Fatty fish such as mackerel and salmon contain omega-3 fatty acids, a type of fat that in large amounts seems to reduce blood pressure. But in at least one study, people with mild high blood pressure who took six grams of fish oil per day for 12 weeks found that their blood pressure sank on average two to four points. The National Heart, Lung and Blood Institute recommends that you chow down on fatty fish as often as possible. If the fish is not fried, the added fat isn't a harmful addition to your total fat budget,

addition to putting folks on medication, many doctors consistently gave just one piece of advice to people whose blood pressure exceeded 140 over 90: "Ditch the salt."

"It's tough to get a consensus in this area, because the effects of sodium chloride on blood pressure are quite complex," says Dr. McCarron. "But our lab has found that people who experience a rise in blood pressure when they take sodium chloride are probably responding to sodium only in the absence of potassium, calcium and magnesium."

"In other words, too much salt is not and never has been

---

since it would likely replace unhealthy saturated fats.

NIX THE DRINKS. The effect of alcohol on blood pressure is so strong that some researchers believe it accounts for up to 5 percent of all high blood pressure. Among 58,218 nurses who were 39 to 59 years old at the start of a four-year study, Harvard researchers found that those who drank two or three alcoholic beverages daily increased their risk of high blood pressure by 40 percent. The National Heart, Lung and Blood Institute suggests that, if you drink, limit it to two drinks or fewer a day.

DON'T WORRY ABOUT CAFFEINE. Caffeine in coffee, tea and sodas only makes blood pressure go up for a few minutes in most people. So unless your doctor tells you otherwise, don't worry about it.

CUT DOWN ON SUGAR. "Work from my laboratory shows that sugar—the kind in your sugar bowl or in foods—raises blood pressure," says Harry Preuss, M.D., professor of medicine at Georgetown University School of Medicine in Washington, D.C. Researchers don't yet know how much sugar it takes to cause a problem. "But it's always a good idea to limit sugar," Dr. Preuss advises.

what jacks up your blood pressure," says Dr. McCarron. The problem is just as likely to be too little potassium, calcium and magnesium.

The Misunderstood Mineral

In retrospect, it's not hard to understand how doctors misread the effects of sodium chloride on blood pressure.

Nobody knew what caused most cases of high blood pressure. So in trying to figure what sends it through the roof, scientists conducted a series of studies in which they took blood pressure readings on a group of people, asked them about what they did or didn't eat, then ran the answers through a computer. The results seemed to indicate that people who used a lot of salt frequently had slightly higher blood pressure readings. Actually, people who used salt heavily had nearly the same blood pressure readings as those who tended to restrict their salt intake. In fact, so many heavy salt users placed on a very low salt diet remained unaffected—up to 67 percent in one study—that researchers began to wonder if some people were "salt-sensitive" while others weren't.

Some people are, says Dr. McCarron. "But," he adds, "it's more likely a relative deficiency of other minerals in the diet—potassium, calcium and magnesium—that determines who is and who is not."

How is he so sure?

Part of the answer is that putting people on low-salt diets has not had the extensive impact on reducing the health consequences of high blood pressure that scientists expected.

In a study at the Medical University–Polyclinic in Bonn, Germany, researchers put 147 men and women between the ages of 19 and 78 with normal blood pressure on a salt-restricted diet—1,000 milligrams, or less than ¼ teaspoon a day—for seven days, then compared their blood pressure levels to a seven-day high-salt diet with over 15,000 milligrams or 3 teaspoons a day. They found that a salt-restricted diet did, in fact, lower blood pressure 17 percent.

But blood pressure during the salt-resticted diet remained

largely unaffected in 67 percent of the people, and it went up in 16 percent. What's more, low-density lipoprotein (LDL) cholesterol levels—the "bad" cholesterol that sets the stage for heart disease and stroke—went up significantly.

The bottom line? A low-salt diet did *not* appear to lower blood pressure in approximately 80 percent of those in the German study. Instead, this research showed that it may be just as likely to raise blood pressure as lower it in people with normal blood pressure—plus it may raise LDL cholesterol levels enough to increase the risk of heart disease. Other studies have shown that salt-restricted diets may have no effect on about two-thirds of people with mild high blood pressure, and less than 25 percent get any noticeable reduction in blood pressure. Indeed, low-salt diets were found to raise blood pressure for nearly 15 percent of people with high blood pressure.

In fact, that could be why a study at the Albert Einstein College of Medicine and Cornell University Medical College in New York City showed that men who ate the least salt each day (about five grams, or one teaspoon) are four times more likely to have a heart attack—the very health consequence a low-salt diet is supposed to prevent—than those who ate more than twice as much salt every day. While too few women were studied to draw a firm conclusion, the researchers observed that the same pattern may be the case for women, too.

It just doesn't make sense that sodium—a mineral that the body requires to survive—could be so harmful, says Dr. McCarron. "There's a biological need for sodium chloride," he explains. "In my view, people appear to need about 3,000 to 4,000 milligrams in their diets on a day-to-day basis in order to maintain optimal blood pressure control. Without any salt at all, your blood pressure would be very low and you could lose consciousness."

"You even have physiological mechanisms—whole systems of hormones—to conserve sodium chloride because it's so necessary," says Dr. McCarron. These systems wouldn't have evolved unless you needed the nutrient, he explains. Nor would the amount of salt that people eat remain relatively constant from person to person—even across international borders. Although some folks have tried to blame processed foods such as lunchmeat and fast-food megaburgers for the roughly 3,300 milligrams of salt most of us eat every day, the truth is that people eat pretty much the same amount of salt no matter what foods are commonly consumed. "Some reports show that the average American salt intake hasn't changed much since the 1870s—well before canned soups or fast-food restaurants" says Dr. McCarron.

"Every scientific survey—and not just in the United States, but also in Mexico, Europe, Canada and Asia—shows that there is a very tight clustering of the population's sodium intake," says Dr. McCarron. "Every group of people takes in between 3,200 and 4,500 milligrams of sodium."

The fact is that "if you turn the human animal loose on this planet to forage for food, for whatever reason, that's the intake they seek," he says.

The Power of Potassium

Although the body clearly needs a certain amount of salt to maintain blood pressure, it also needs certain levels of potassium, calcium and magnesium. These minerals can help keep sodium levels in the body from getting too high, explains Dr. McCarron.

"While there's no fixed recommendation for potassium," he says, "most researchers agree that we should have between 3,000 to 3,200 milligrams a day."

But does that level lower blood pressure?

Yes. In a three-week study of 87 African-American men and women at the Johns Hopkins Medical Institutions in Baltimore, researchers took blood pressure measurements, divided the group in half, then gave potassium supplements of 3,120 milligrams a day to one group and a placebo to the other.

The result? Systolic blood pressure—the top number of your blood pressure reading—went down an average of 6.9 points in people who received the supplements, while diastolic pressure—the bottom number—went down an average of 2.5 points. There were no blood pressure changes in the group that took the placebo.

No one really knows exactly how potassium lowers blood pressure, reports Frederick L. Brancati, M.D., assistant professor of medicine and epidemiology, who led the study. One theory suggests that potassium relaxes small blood vessels, while another suggests that it helps the body eliminate water and salt.

Since most folks only get around 2,600 milligrams of the nutrient a day, however, Dr. McCarron suggests that most of us need to add at least three servings of potassium-rich fresh fruits and vegetables, such as bananas and potatoes, as well as dairy products—a glass of milk has nearly as much potassium as a banana—to our diets every day.

Magnesium's Magic

Along with potassium, magnesium seems to play an important role in keeping blood pressure down—particularly if

Prescription for Healing

Several nutrients may play a role in keeping a lid on blood pressure. Here are the amounts that researchers recommend you get, first from dietary sources, then a multivitamin supplement if necessary.

NUTRIENT	DAILY AMOUNT
Potassium	3,000 to 3,200 milligrams
Magnesium	300 to 400 milligrams
Calcium	1,000 milligrams (men 25 to 65)
	1,500 milligrams (men over 65)
	1,000 milligrams (women 25 to 50 or on estrogen replacement therapy)
	1,500 milligrams (women over 65 or pregnant or postmenopausal and not on estrogens)
Vitamin C	240 milligrams

you're magnesium-deficient to begin with.

In a study in Sweden of 71 people with mildly elevated blood pressure, researchers found that giving about 350 milligrams of magnesium to those who had a magnesium deficiency lowered their blood pressure readings several points.

How does it work in people with high blood pressure who may not have a deficiency?

Some studies indicate that it won't do much of anything, although at least one indicates that it might. That study, conducted by researchers in Belgium and the Netherlands, looked at the blood pressure levels of 47 women with high blood pressure. When researchers gave the women 485 milligrams of magnesium every day for six months, the top number on the women's blood pressure readings dropped an average of 2.7 points, while the bottom number dropped 3.4 points. A few of the women had low levels of magnesium in their blood, but most did not. That drop doesn't sound like a lot. But to someone with borderline high blood pressure, it can mean the difference between taking medication and eating salmon, which is rich magnesium.

Most people should get between 300 and 400 milligrams of magnesium daily to keep their blood pressure on an even keel, says Dr. McCarron. Currently, only adult males in the United States get the full amount. Women between 30 and 60 years old get between 220 and 260 milligrams a day. Good food sources for magnesium are green leafy vegetables, fish, whole grains and rice, legumes and nuts.

Calcium for Kids and Moms

Although some studies on calcium and blood pressure have indicated that calcium might play a role in keeping blood pressure under control, a panel of experts at the National Institutes of Health in Bethesda, Maryland, has determined that most studies indicate that its role is probably minor, and a recommendation to increase calcium intake for blood pressure control is unwarranted at this time for most people.

"The two exceptions may be in pregnant women who have high blood pressure during pregnancy and in children who are calcium-deficient," says Matthew W. Gillman, M.D., assistant professor of ambulatory care and prevention at Harvard Medical School, who has investigated the relationship between calcium and blood pressure.

In a study at the University of Florida Health Science Center in Jacksonville, for example, researchers found that 2,000 milligrams of calcium a day reduced the onset of high blood pressure in women during pregnancy by 54 percent.

Until scientists more clearly define who calcium does and does not help, however, everyone should make sure he gets the optimal Daily Value (DV), says Dr. McCarron.

The National Institutes of Health recommend that the optimal daily intake is 1,000 milligrams for men ages 25 to 65 and 1,500 milligrams for men over 65. The Institutes recommend 1,000 milligrams daily for women between the ages of 25 and 50 and women on estrogen replacement therapy, and 1,500 milligrams for pregnant women, postmenopausal women not taking estrogen replacements and women over 65. These recommendations are in line with the DV for calcium of 1,000 milligrams.

Unfortunately, federal surveys indicate that women ages 25 to 50 get only between 685 and 778 milligrams a day through their daily diets. Women over 50 get between 600 and 700 milligrams. Adult men get closer to the mark, generally getting between 700 and 1,000 milligrams.

A Role for Vitamin C

A number of studies indicate that vitamin C may also be involved in reducing blood pressure.

In analyzing the results of four separate studies conducted at Tufts University in Boston, researchers found that the less vitamin C in the diet, the higher your blood pressure is likely to be.

In one of these studies, researchers found that some individuals consuming 240 milligrams a day or more of vitamin C were 50 percent less likely to have high blood pressure than those who consumed less than 60 milligrams a day.

New studies that will test whether or not adding vitamin

C to a diet can actually lower blood pressure are under way. In the meantime, the level of vitamin C used in the Tufts study—in the neighborhood of 240 milligrams a day—is considered safe, says Dr. McCarron. (Although the DV for vitamin C is only 60 milligrams, consuming 240 milligrams every day is well within the safe limits for vitamin C.)

Zinc and Other Immune Sparkers
Say So Long to Yeast Infections

HAVE ITCHY PALMS? Some would say that money's coming your way. A seven-year itch? Better have a heart-felt chat with your mate. An itch where, well, you'd rather not discuss it? Welcome to one of the most common of feminine struggles: woman versus the beast called yeast.

In fact, at some point during their childbearing years, three out of four women will wonder what they did to deserve the itching, burning, odor and unpleasant discharge that accompany vaginal yeast infections. They'll also want to know what exactly they can do to stop it from ever happening again.

Yeast-Fighting Basics

Fortunately, there are steps women can take to prevent these itchy episodes, but first it helps to understand why a yeast infection happens at all.

The most likely culprit behind this maddening malady is a generally mild-mannered fungus known as *Candida albicans* that lives in the vagina, mouth and intestines. Normally, candida is kept to its small, harmless colonies by the immune system and by *Lactobacillus acidophilus*—another bacteria commonly found in the vagina that creates an acidic environment that candida don't like. When something throws this ecosystem off balance, however, candida run rampant and yeast infections can result.

The most common offenders—things that upset this delicate ecosystem—include wet bathing suits, panty hose, skin-tight jeans and leotards. All of these things foster a warm, moist environment that candida love. Women are also prone to yeast infections during pregnancy, just before they get their periods and during menopause. Candida also multiply when women take antibiotics, because such medications often kill too many good bacteria, such as *Lactobacilli*, along with the bad, leaving candida unchecked.

Be a Bad Host with Good Nutrition

Once candida has spread to a flaming yeast infection, doctor's commonly recommend over-the-counter medications such as miconazole (Monistat), clotrimazole (Gyne-Lotrimin) or the new one-dose, prescription-only fluconazole (Diflucan), all of which can have you sitting comfortably again in less than a week. But since these medications won't kick candida out for good, and yeast infection recurrence is common, doctors say that you have to be a bad host if you want to remain yeast-free.

"Treating the vagina alone is often a waste of time and money," says William Crook, M.D., a physician in private practice in Jackson, Tennessee, and author of *The Yeast Connection and the Woman*. "Although vaginal suppositories may help, we also need to concentrate on putting the right things in your body to take care of the source of the problem."

According to the experts, that means boosting your immunity through a good diet and nutritional supplements such as vitamins C, E, A and the mineral zinc. Here's what they recommend.

Note: Although *Candida albicans* is the most common cause of vaginal infection, it isn't the only cause. So if you've never had a yeast infection before, see your doctor for a proper diagnosis before starting any treatment on your own.

Build Immunity with Zinc

When it comes to disease fighting, the trace mineral zinc is often a heavyweight contender. It stimulates the production of T lymphocyte cells—the cells in your immune system responsible for cleaning up cells that have been invaded by infection. According to medical research, this makes zinc a prize fighter against *Candida albicans.*

In fact, zinc supplements are likely beneficial even if you're body's zinc levels are normal, according to a study done in India. Researchers there worked with laboratory animals that were *not* deficient in zinc. They gave these animals high-dose zinc supplements and found that they were significantly more

Yogurt, Yes; Sugar, No

You probably already know that shedding a wet bathing suit or sweaty underclothing is good prevention against moisture-loving yeast infections. But you might not know that doctors have found that adding or subtracting certain foods from your diet might help fight these itchy occurrences as well. Here are their dietary recommendations for staying yeast-free.

SAY YES TO YOGURT. Whoever developed the old home remedy of douching with yogurt to stop a yeast infection was close to being right—she was just putting it in the wrong place! You have to eat it—a cup a day—and it has to contain active *Lactobacillus acidophilus* cultures. (If the yogurt contains live cultures, it will say so on the label.)

In a study of 33 women at the Long Island Jewish Medical Center, researchers found that women with a history of yeast infection recurrence could decrease the incidence of recurrence threefold just by eating eight ounces of yogurt a day.

SAY NO TO SWEETS. *Candida albicans* (the med-

resistant to infection from *Candida albicans* than those not supplemented with zinc.

"Zinc is essential in preventing infection," agrees Dr. Crook. "And though it's best to get your vitamins and minerals through a healthy diet, given how many essential nutrients our food loses by the time it's processed, packaged, shipped and bought, supplementation is probably a good idea."

To fight candida, Tori Hudson, M.D., professor at the National College for Naturopathic Medicine in Portland, Oregon, suggests taking 15 milligrams (the Daily Value, or DV) of zinc. And to get more zinc through your diet, try oysters. They contain more than 76 milligrams per half-dozen.

---

ical term for the kind of yeast that causes vaginal infection) is a fungus with a real sweet tooth. Indulging in too many sweet, sugary foods can raise your blood glucose and create the perfect candida breeding ground, according to William Crook, M.D., a physician in private practice in Jackson, Tennessee, and author of *The Yeast Connection and the Woman*.

SKIP YEASTY FOODS. Though there hasn't been any research to confirm this, some doctors report that women prone to yeast infections can experience outbreaks from eating yeasty foods. Dr. Crook suggests avoiding foods such as pizza and beer as well as aged foods such as wine, cheese and smoked meats.

COOK WITH GARLIC. Garlic contains an anti-microbial agent known as allicin. There is some evidence that candida simply hate garlic. Some women find that eating a clove of garlic a day helps prevent yeast infection, says Tori Hudson, M.D., professor at the National College for Naturopathic Medicine in Portland, Oregon.

Fight Infection with C

When it comes to fighting *Candida albicans*, Vitamin C is a double-action agent.

First, research has shown that it boosts immunity by keeping the disease-fighting white blood cells up and running so that the body is better able to stave off infections, especially "opportunistic" ones such as candida that take advantage of a weak immune system.

As a bonus, vitamin C adds acidic zip to your vaginal environment. "Candida-fighting *Lactobacillus* grows in acid," explains Roy M. Pitkin, M.D., professor of obstetrics and gynecology at the University of California, Los Angeles, "so taking vitamin C may help, though it isn't likely to be completely effective by itself."

For optimum results, Dr. Hudson recommends 4,000 milligrams of vitamin C a day, divided into two 2,000-milligram doses—once in the morning and once in the evening for "better absorption."

This amount is considerably higher than the DV for vitamin C, which is only 60 milligrams. Although these high amounts of vitamin C are considered safe, some people may experience diarrhea from amounts over 1,000 milligrams. If you want to try these higher doses to prevent yeast infection, discuss it with your doctor.

Think fruits and vegetables if you want to turn up the level of vitamin C in your diet. One cup of broccoli, orange juice or brussels sprouts provides about 100 milligrams.

Scare Yeast Away with A and E

For women who have an ongoing battle with candida, Dr. Hudson also recommends adding two more immunity-boosting vitamins to the mix—A and E.

"Vitamin A can be used either of two ways," says Dr. Hudson. Women can take vitamin A supplements of 25,000 international units (IU) a day (a dose that is 20,000 IU above the DV and should be monitored by your doctor). Or, if they prefer not to take such high amounts orally, women can insert the vitamin into the vagina instead.

"Inserting vitamin A stimulates the immune system right in the vagina," says Dr. Hudson. "You can simply insert a vitamin A gelatin capsule, although they are less potent than the vitamin A suppositories made by several companies."

As a final precautionary measure, she recommends taking 400 IU of vitamin E.

If you're a frequent victim of the yeast beast and would like to increase these nutrients in your diet, try cooking with vegetable oils and eating whole-grain cereals for more vitamin E, drinking fortified skim milk for a burst of vitamin A and upping your intake of bright orange vegetables to increase beta-carotene (a substance that turns to vitamin A in the body).

Keeping Yeast at Bay

While medicated creams will give your most tender areas the quickest relief from an annoying yeast infection, you'll need some nutritional immunity builders if you want to prevent recurrence. Here's what experts suggest.

NUTRIENT	AMOUNT
Zinc	15 milligrams a day
Vitamin C*	2,000 milligrams twice a day
Vitamin A†	25,000 IU a day (or a gelatin capsule as a suppository)
Vitamin E	400 IU a day

*The Daily Value for Vitamin C is only 60 milligrams. While higher amounts are considered safe, some people experience diarrhea from taking just 1,000 milligrams. So check with your doctor before trying these higher doses.

†Vitamin A can be toxic in high doses. Check with your doctor before exceeding 15,000 IU a day.

Part IV

Prevention Cuisine:
Low-Fat at Its Best

Your Supermarket Survival Guide

Lean, Mean Heart-Smart Cuisine

As you may already know, doctors recommend a diet that derives no more than 25 percent of its total calories from fat. But you can't put low-fat foods on your table if you don't put them in your shopping cart first. And that may not seem easy at first glance: Instead of limiting your reading to price tags, you'll have to scan labels on food packaging as well. But don't despair. Reading labels really isn't so tough, and the rewards are significant: fewer doctor visits and a longer life span, not to mention a trimmer form.

Ready to begin your quest for low-fat fare? Read on for tips on what to toss in your cart.

Stick to the Basics

In general, you'll find the healthiest and least expensive fare around the perimeter of the supermarket—fresh produce, lean meats and fish and low-fat and nonfat dairy products. The inner aisles contain some low-fat foods, such as pasta, beans and grains. But you'll have to read labels to make sure that other inner-aisle products, such as cake mixes, canned soups and frozen dinners, fill the low-fat bill.

While you're checking out the fat content of those pre-pared foods, look at their sugar and sodium contents, too: Many prepackaged foods have little fat but lots of sugar and/or sodium. If diabetes or high blood pressure runs in your family (or if you already have either condition), ask your doctor about ways you should modify your diet for optimal health.

It's also wise to remember that man (and woman) cannot live on convenience foods alone—they're too expensive and not nearly as healthful as a diet of fresh fruits and vegetables, grains and low-fat meats. Here, then, is a guide to choosing the lowest-fat produce, baked goods, deli items, poultry and seafood.

The produce aisle. On the whole, you can feel free to load up your cart with the healthful, low-fat and vitamin-rich fresh foods in this aisle. But beware of those prepackaged "companion foods" that grocers slip in among the healthful fare— the bacon bits, fatty cream dressings and caramel apple dips you'll find here usually have lots of fat and/or calories. And don't go too nuts over almonds, sunflower seeds or avocados,

Fat Math 101

Does that cereal, cheese or frozen entrée meet your low-fat needs? You can find out by doing a few simple calculations. Here's how.

1. Look on the product's "Nutrition Facts" label for the number of fat grams per serving. One gram of fat has 9 calories. So to get the number of calories from fat, then multiply the food's total fat grams per serving by 9.

2. Find the product's total calories per serving. Divide the number you just computed by the total calories per serving. Then multiply the result by 100, and you have the percent of calories from fat.

Here's an example of "fat math" in action. A ¾-cup serving of Apple-Cinnamon Cheerios contains 2.5 grams of fat. Multiplying 2.5 fat grams times 9 calories per gram of fat equals 22.5 calories from fat. The total calories per ¾ cup of this cereal is 120. Dividing 22.5 by 120 equals 0.1875. Multiply that by 100, and your percentage of calories from fat equals about 19—well within the acceptable range.

either: While they're great sources of vitamin E, they're also high in fat.

The bakery. Bread has always been a relatively low-fat food, and now the shelves are stocked with fat-free and low-fat prepackaged versions. If you're buying fresh-baked breads and desserts from the grocery's bakery, however, you won't know the fat content of the goods unless you ask. And chances are, the person behind the counter won't know the answer.

To be on the safe side, treat fresh-baked goods as occasional indulgences and look for whole-grain varieties made without partially or fully hydrogenated oils.

The deli. This section can be trouble if you don't choose wisely. Some delis offer nutritional information on their homemade dishes (like ravioli, macaroni salad and baked beans), but many don't. If you can't get reliable info, it's best to invest in a cookbook with low-fat recipes and whip up your own deli-style delights.

As for lunchmeats, forget about taking a number and choose from the wide variety of prepackaged low-fat (and sometimes low-sodium) lunchmeats. If you prefer fresh-sliced deli meats, ask the counter person to tell you the specific fat content of meats that claim to be low in fat. You'll want products with no more than one gram of fat per ounce. (The wrapper should be labeled—you just have to persuade the counter person to show it to you.) The lowest-fat choices are usually sliced turkey or chicken breast. Most delis also offer a few types of low-fat cheese but, again, ask the counter person if you can see the label.

The meat, poultry and seafood counters. Unless you have doctor's orders to the contrary, you can occasionally have a little red meat or pork. Choose the leanest cuts and trim off all visible fat. And eat small portions of red meat—no more than four to six ounces a day.

At the beef counter, choose cuts from the loin or round (leg) that are marked "select," the grade that contains the least fat. Also, take care to choose only the leanest ground round: The more specks of white in the meat, the fattier it is. Pork fans should select tenderloin or loin chops.

When choosing poultry, remember that white meat (breast meat) is leanest, followed by thigh meat and then the meat on wings and drumsticks. You can cook the poultry in its skin to keep the meat moist, but remove the fat and skin before serving. If you're buying ground chicken or turkey, select ground breast meat; packages labeled "ground turkey" or "ground chicken" may contain fattier leg meat and skin as well as breast meat.

Eight Ways to Defat Your Food Bill

Here are eight quick tips to help you trim the fat from your grocery bill—and your groceries.

1. Make a list and stick to it.

2. Watch for sales, but don't buy something fatty just because it's cheap. You'll pay for it later—with your health.

3. Use coupons whenever possible. But weed out the ones for high-fat items so you won't be tempted to purchase them.

4. Buy fruits and vegetables in season. The fresher the produce, the higher the nutrient content.

5. Buy store brands instead of name brands. Just be sure to read the product labels for fat, sodium and sugar content.

6. Avoid buying processed foods.

7. Use low-fat recipes to prepare foods such as soups, stews and desserts at home, then freeze leftovers. This is cheaper than buying premade frozen dinners and desserts. It's healthier, too, because you avoid chemical additives and preservatives.

8. When there's a sale, stock up on nonperishable products like frozen veggies and canned or dried beans.

Even the fattiest fish is lower in fat and cholesterol than most meats, so seafood's always a good choice. What's more, its fat is generally the heart-healthy omega-3 kind, which has been shown to lower total cholesterol levels, increase levels of high-density lipoprotein, or HDL, cholesterol (the kind that helps keep arteries free and clear) and decrease the risk of heart disease. Haddock, flounder, cod and clams are among the lowest-fat varieties, as is yellowfin tuna. Atlantic salmon and mackerel sport high levels of omega-3's.

While the type of meats, poultry and fish you choose is important, cooking these items healthfully is equally important. That means stir-frying chicken in a teaspoon of oil instead of deep-frying it or steaming or baking fish rather than broiling it in butter.

Greens, Glorious Greens
Add Sizzle to Your Salad Days

AT *PREVENTION* MAGAZINE WE THINK you can never get enough glorious greens no matter how, or even if, you cook them. That's because the more you eat of them, the better off you are. Greens, collectively, are the one food you can love that loves you right back. Chicory, Swiss chard, kale, dandelion, radicchio . . . the list goes on and on.

To some people these words may seem like part of a foreign-language primer, but don't let strange-sounding names put you off. We realize that even though you know deep down these curious vegetables are great for you, they may be somewhat intimidating at first.

So we'll take it slow and introduce you to a few of these green giants, sort of glossary-style, and show you there's a whole spectrum of delicious greens just waiting to be explored!

Meet the Green Team

All the greens in this chapter are readily available in most supermarkets; just take a stroll down the emerald aisle. You'll find these greens are great in salads, soups and stews. Or simply add a splash of olive oil or citrus juice and a sprinkle of Parmesan or chopped nuts (see cooking suggestions on page 252) and enjoy!

Note: Nutritional analyses for the following vegetables are based on a one-cup serving, raw.

Kale. Thick, handsomely ruffled, grayish blue to green, kale is perhaps the most misunderstood green. It's often called upon to act as window dressing at salad bars, probably because it stays fresh so long when perched on a bed of crushed ice. But boasting a mild cabbagelike flavor, kale is as versatile as spinach. Avoid yellowed leaves. It's available year-round and the season peaks January through April.

Nutrient profile: A member of the Crucifer family. High in vitamin C (80 milligrams), potassium (299 milligrams), beta-carotene (3.58 milligrams) and calcium (90 milligrams); 33 calories.

Tip: With kale, looks are everything. Choose leaves with good, green color and a crisp, moist, clean, cold appearance. And remember: The darker green the leaf, the higher the nutritional value.

Dandelion greens. These bright green, jagged-edged leaves have a strong, tart flavor. They grow both wild (in your own backyard!) and cultivated. The peak season is early spring, before plants begin to develop their infamous yellow flowers. At this point the leaves become tough and bitter. Look for bright green, tender-crisp leaves with no yellowing or wilted tips.

Nutrient profile: Excellent source of beta-carotene (4.6 milligrams) and calcium (103 milligrams) and a good source of vitamin C (19 milligrams) and iron; 24 calories.

Tip: Handle greens with TLC. Cuts and bruises invite decay.

Swiss chard. These fleshy, silvery, celery stalk–like stems have broad, crisp, crinkly green leaves. The sturdy stems are often used like celery or asparagus in cooking. Swiss chard leaves, with their sweet, earthy taste and slightly bitter undertone, can be cooked like any other green. The peak season is April through November.

Nutrient profile: Chard boasts 11 milligrams of vitamin C and is a source of magnesium; only 6 calories.

Tip: Always steam chard—boiling removes the flavor.

Beet greens. These are actually the green tops of the beet root vegetable and may be sold attached to full-size beets or in bunches by themselves. The long-stemmed green or greenish red leaves are significantly more nutritious than their ruby-red roots. Beet greens are best when they're young. They're available year-round and the peak season is June through October.

Nutrient profile: 1.4 milligrams beta-carotene, 45 milligrams calcium, 1.4 grams fiber, 11 milligrams vitamin C; 7 calories.

Tip: Be forewarned—beet greens tend to bleed when cooked and will impart a red color if added to soups.

Mustard greens. These are thinner and softer in texture than most varieties of greens, with a tempting, tangy mustard flavor. Look for crisp, young leaves with a bright green color. Avoid yellow, flabby or pitted leaves, greens with mustard seeds attached (a sign of overmaturity) or thick, fibrous stems. The peak season is December through early March.

Nutrient profile: A member of the Crucifer family. Good source of vitamin C (39 milligrams), folacin (105 micrograms) and calcium (58 milligrams); only 15 calories.

Tip: The volume of these greens reduces drastically during cooking, so be sure to prepare enough. One pound raw equals one cup cooked.

Turnip greens. Slightly sweet when young and tender, turnip greens become tough and strong-flavored with age. Buy only fresh, green, even-colored crisp turnip tops; avoid those that are wilted or off-color. Prepare like spinach. The peak season is October through February.

Nutrient profile: 105 milligrams calcium, 107 micrograms folacin, 33 milligrams vitamin C, 2.5 milligrams beta-carotene; only 15 calories.

Tip: Don't store greens in the same refrigerator drawer as you do ethylene-producing fruits such as apples; the greens will develop brown spots and decay rapidly.

Spinach. Good spinach has a musky flavor with a coarse texture. Look for fresh, crisp, dark green outer leaves that are free of dirt and debris. Inner leaves will be pale, crinkled and very tender. Wimpy, wilted, limp and brownish leaves have lost vitamin C. Spinach is superb raw or cooked. Lightly steamed fresh spinach has excellent flavor and texture. But fresh, perky raw spinach shines in a salad alone or is very compatible with other greens. Try it with fruits such as strawberries

Clean Greens Are Happy Greens

Clean your greens as soon as you whisk them home from market, especially if they're wet (wet leaves tend to rot easily). Here's how.

• Discard the tatty, imperfect leaves. Break whole heads apart and remove thick stems, such as those on spinach.

• Fill your sink or a large bowl with cold water. Add the leaves and swish them around with your hands to dislodge dirt and grit. But don't soak: Soaking dissolves some of the valuable nutrients. Change the water once or twice if the leaves are especially dirty. Transfer to a colander and give the leaves a final cold-water rinse.

• If you are cooking the greens immediately, give them a slight shake, but allow some water droplets to remain for more even cooking.

• If you plan to store your greens, dry them well between paper or cotton toweling or use a salad spinner.

• Store in plastic bags that have been perforated for air circulation. Close securely, refrigerate and use within three to four days.

or mandarin oranges, a few red onion slices and a splash of olive oil. Outstanding! Spinach is available year-round.

Nutrient profile: Contains a lusty 109 micrograms of folacin, 44 milligrams magnesium, 312 milligrams potassium, 16 milligrams vitamin C; only 14 calories.

Tip: Spinach has stamina. When stored at 34° to 36°F with a relative humidity of 90 to 95 percent, spinach says fresh for at least 10 to 14 days.

Chicory greens. Also known as curly endive, these greens have a pleasantly bitter taste. Look for narrow leaves that have a curly edge and are curling at the ends. The center should be yellowish white with darker outer leaves that are tender and crisp with no signs of wilting. Chicory greens are available year-round. Radicchio is a red-leafed Italian chicory.

Nutrient profile: Chicory tops the green scene as an excellent source of vitamin C (43 milligrams), calcium (180 milligrams), folacin (197 milligrams), magnesium (54 milligrams) and potassium (756 milligrams); 41 calories.

Tip: Use a light touch when cooking these greens; otherwise you'll lose some valuable water-soluble nutrients and texture.

Gussy Up Those Greens

You probably think that if you've tried one green, you've tried them all. *Au contraire!* While it's true that most greens are interchangeable in recipes, their characteristics vary greatly. And a lot hinges on how you prepare them and with what. Don't forget, creative seasoning packs greens with fantastic flavor, not fat. So turn over a new leaf and veer away from buttery, creamy sauces; stick to gourmet seasoning mixes and follow these cooking suggestions for some groovy green grazing.

Wilting. Here's an easy way to wilt greens with no added fat. To wilt greens with a small amount of fat, follow the directions below. But in step 2 add a small amount of olive oil to the pan. When the oil is hot, add some chopped garlic and sauté until golden.

1. Clean the greens (see "Clean Greens Are Happy Greens" on page 251) and have them ready in a colander. Don't shake off all the water, though; it helps to steam the greens.
2. Heat a large, no-stick frying pan over medium to high heat.
3. Add the wet greens (you have to begin with a mountain of greens; 1 pound raw equals 1 cup cooked) to the hot pan and cook, covered, over medium-high heat until wilted and bright green. This procedure takes only a few minutes. Serve over pasta with a dollop of plain nonfat yogurt mixed with horseradish and chives.

Braising. If your greens are tough and strong, take the wilting procedure one step further. After the greens have wilted in the pan, stir in a little stock or water, cover, reduce the heat to medium-low and cook a bit longer. After about 5 minutes, taste and be your own judge. Drizzle some lemon juice or apple cider over the greens before serving.

As a bonus, the gentle braising method produces a delicious "pot liquor"—the liquid in the pan. Serve with a hunk of crunchy French bread for sopping up every last drop.

Microwaving. Toss fresh, chopped greens into a glass dish. Splash on some stock and cover with vented plastic wrap. Microwave on high until just tender (about 2 minutes for 2 cups of greens). Allow to stand for 2 minutes, then drain. Add to casseroles, stir-fries and rice dishes or serve simply and elegantly with a sprinkling of Parmesan or feta cheese and chopped nuts.

Blanching. This term means to boil briefly, then cool quickly in cold water. (See the recipe for "Cabbage-Salmon Rolls" on page 258.)

....

Cabbage-Patch Cuisine
Rev Up Your Immune System

IF YOU WERE A TYPICAL KID, chances are you turned up your nose at cabbage. But as an adult, you know how delicious this versatile vegetable can be.

The three primary varieties of cabbage are green, red and savoy. The green and red varieties, available year-round, are ideal in soups, salads and entrées. The more loose-leafed savoy cabbage, which has a webbed texture, is excellent for stuffing but can be hard to find in the dead of winter.

But no matter which variety of cabbage you use, one thing's for sure: You're treating yourself to a mother lode of vitamin C, an antioxidant vitamin thought to help thwart cancer and heart disease. Read on for some of the freshest—and healthiest—ways to prepare cabbage, including a cheesy cabbage bake and a tempting pasta dish.

PASTA AND CABBAGE BOLOGNESE
∽

In this dish, C stands for creative, vitamin C and cabbage—a terrific combination! Best of all, the flavor is high and the fat is low.

    ½ pound extra-lean ground beef
    ½ teaspoon olive oil
    ½ cup chopped onions
    2 cloves garlic, minced
    1 tablespoon snipped fresh basil or ¾ teaspoon dried
    ¼ teaspoon dried oregano
    ½ teaspoon ground black pepper
    ⅛ teaspoon crushed red-pepper flakes

2 teaspoons low-sodium soy sauce

I cup reduced-fat beef broth

I can (16 ounces) crushed tomatoes

8 ounces spaghetti, cooked

3 cups shredded cabbage, steamed

2 tablespoons grated Parmesan cheese

Coat a large frying pan with no-stick spray. Add the beef to the pan and sauté over medium heat until the meat is browned, about 5 minutes. Using a slotted spoon, remove the meat to a plate and set aside. Wipe the pan clean with paper towels.

Add the oil to the pan. Add the onions, garlic, basil, oregano, black pepper, pepper flakes and soy sauce. Sauté, stirring, for 2 to 3 minutes. Add the broth and tomatoes. Bring to a gentle simmer and cook for 5 minutes. Reduce the heat to low and stir in the meat. Cook for 20 minutes, stirring occasionally.

In a large bowl, toss the hot spaghetti, cabbage and Parmesan together. Top with the meat sauce.

Variation: Replace the spaghetti with linguine and the Parmesan with Asiago.

MAKES 4 SERVINGS

 Nutritional Information

Per serving: 308 calories, 3.2 g. fat (9% of calories), 5 mg. cholesterol, 545 mg. sodium, 3.5 g. dietary fiber.

CABBAGE AU GRATIN

∽

The milk and cheese in this dish contribute to your calcium intake.

  1 small head cabbage, halved
2½ teaspoons olive oil
1½ tablespoons flour
  1 cup evaporated skim milk
  ¼ teaspoon black pepper
  ¼ teaspoon ground red pepper
1½ teaspoons snipped fresh sage or ¾ teaspoons dried
  ½ cup shredded fat-free Cheddar cheese
  1 cup fresh bread crumbs
  1 teaspoon paprika

Place the cabbage halves in an 8-quart pot with 2 quarts of boiling water. Cook, uncovered, for 5 minutes. Using a slotted spoon, transfer the cabbage to a colander to drain. Let the water from cooking the cabbage cool.

In a medium saucepan, combine 2 teaspoons of the oil and the flour. Place on low heat and add the milk, 1 cup of the cabbage water, black pepper, red pepper and sage. Cook, stirring constantly, until the sauce thickens, about 3 minutes. Add the Cheddar and cook, stirring, until the cheese melts, about 3 minutes. Remove the cheese sauce from the heat and set aside.

Squeeze the cabbage to remove excess water. Quarter each half, forming four wedges. Coat a shallow 1½-quart casserole with no-stick spray and add the cabbage, flat sides down. Pour the cheese sauce over the cabbage.

Toss the bread crumbs in the remaining ½ teaspoon oil and scatter them over top of the cabbage. Sprinkle with the paprika. Bake at 375° until the crumbs are lightly browned and the cabbage is tender, about 20 minutes.

MAKES 4 SERVINGS

 Nutritional Information

Per serving: 187 calories, 4.4 g. fat (20% of calories), 5 mg. cholesterol, 267 mg. sodium, 3.4 g. dietary fiber.

BLACK-EYED-PEAS-AND-CABBAGE SLAW

This slaw packs fiber and flavor; marinate it overnight for maximum zip.

¼ cup cider or wine vinegar

2 tablespoons lemon juice

1 teaspoon low-sodium soy sauce

2 teaspoons mustard

1 tablespoon olive oil

2 cloves garlic, minced

½ teaspoon black pepper

2 tablespoons finely chopped ginger root

2 tablespoons snipped fresh parsley

1 cup dried black-eyed peas, cooked with 1 bay leaf and drained

4 cups finely shredded cabbage

2 carrots, shredded

½ cup chopped scallions

In a large bowl, combine the vinegar, lemon juice, soy sauce, mustard, oil, garlic, pepper, ginger and parsley. Whisk vigorously with a wire whisk or fork until the dressing is emulsified.

If the bay leaf is still in the peas, remove and discard it. Add the peas, cabbage, carrots and scallions to the vinegar dressing. Toss, cover and chill for at least 2 hours.

Variation: Replace the black-eyed peas with pinto or black beans.

MAKES 6 SERVINGS

 Nutritional Information

Per serving: 107 calories, 2.8 g. fat (22% of calories), 0 mg. cholesterol, 80 mg. sodium, 5.5 g. dietary fiber.

CABBAGE-SALMON ROLLS

These delicious roll-ups are a breeze to make.

1 clove garlic, minced

2 plum tomatoes, coarsely chopped, or ½ cup canned tomatoes, chopped

2 teaspoons snipped fresh dill or ½ teaspoon dried

¼ teaspoon black pepper

1 cup clam broth or reduced-fat chicken broth

2 cups cooked brown rice

½ cup chopped scallions

½ cup chopped sweet red peppers

1 teaspoon low-sodium soy sauce

8 cabbage leaves, blanched for 5 minutes

1 pound salmon fillet, cut into 8 equal pieces

In a medium saucepan, combine the garlic, tomatoes, dill, black pepper and clam or chicken broth. Cover the pan and heat the mixture over medium heat for about 5 minutes.

In a medium bowl, combine the rice, scallions, red peppers and soy sauce. Spread about ¼ cup of the rice mixture in the center of each cabbage leaf. Top the rice with a piece of the salmon, then roll each leaf into a tight bundle. Fasten with a toothpick, if necessary. (Remove the toothpicks before serving.)

Place the salmon rolls, seam side down, in a 2-quart casserole. Pour the tomato mixture over the rolls. Cover the casserole with a lid or foil and bake at 400° until the salmon is tender and flaky, about 15 minutes.

MAKES 4 SERVINGS

 Nutritional Information

Per serving: 303 calories, 8.2 g. fat (24% of calories), 61 mg. cholesterol, 199 mg. sodium, 4.1 g. dietary fiber.

MADRAS CABBAGE

ᥬᥩ

A taste of India highlights this recipe. The fat's a tad over our usual 25 percent, but don't worry—it's from the chick-peas, so it's monounsaturated.

1 cup reduced-fat chicken broth

3 teaspoons curry powder (or to taste)

1 teaspoon black pepper

2 tablespoons snipped parsley

1 clove garlic, minced

1 chili pepper, seeded and minced
(wear plastic gloves when handling)

4 carrots, sliced

1 teaspoon olive oil

4 cups shredded cabbage

½ cup chick-peas

In a large saucepan, combine the broth, curry powder, black pepper, parsley, garlic, chili peppers, carrots and oil. Simmer over medium heat for 7 minutes. Stir in the cabbage and cook, covered, until the cabbage is tender, 5 to 7 minutes. Add the chick-peas and heat for 3 minutes.

MAKES 4 SERVINGS

 Nutritional Information

Per serving: 122 calories, 4.2 g. fat (29% of calories), 2 mg. cholesterol, 213 mg. sodium, 5.1 g. dietary fiber.

The Tasty Bean

Going Meatless Can Be Marvelous

Beans are nutritional gems—easy to prepare, inexpensive and widely available. If you are looking for healthful food that tastes good, you've hit the jackpot.

The term "beans" loosely refers to the members of the legume family, which also includes split peas, lentils and peanuts. Legumes come in a multitude of shapes, sizes and colors. There are hundreds of varieties of legumes, from kidney-shaped red and white beans to cream-colored black-eyed peas.

Not too long ago, beans were on the verge of falling into an abyss of obsolete cuisine. But that was then; this is now. Beans are on the rebound and have never been more popular. Supermarkets and natural food stores are expanding shelf space and selling more and more varieties of beans. There is also a growing interest in ethnic cuisines, a traditional haven for bean-inspired dishes.

So if you are striving to eat healthful meals with delicious flavors, you've come to the right place.

A Mother Lode of Nutrients

Beans are a "power food," loaded with nutrients and fiber and low in fat, calories and sodium. Like all food derived from plants, beans have zero cholesterol.

Beans, peas and lentils are a super source of nutrients. They are high in vitamins and minerals, including the B-complex vitamins, iron, calcium, potassium, zinc and magnesium. In addition, beans are the kingpin of protein in the vegetable world. (While the protein is incomplete, when beans are served with rice, tortillas, bread or other cereal grains, the protein is completed.) Beans are also considered a good source of complex carbohydrates. They take a long time to digest, making you feel sated longer.

Dried beans are naturally low in sodium; canned beans tend to contain more sodium. Rinsing the canned beans, however, dramatically reduces the sodium content. Recently, low-sodium canned beans have been showing up on the supermarket shelves.

Beans, peas and lentils are rich in dietary fiber. Also called roughage, fiber is the indigestible part of our food that provides bulk and promotes regularity in our digestive systems. There are two kinds of dietary fiber: insoluble and soluble. Insoluble fiber relieves constipation, and soluble fiber has been shown to decrease blood cholesterol levels. Beans contain both forms of fiber.

Try One . . . or Try Them All

The world of beans is filled with versatile, multicolored, multishaped members. Here are some of the most popular.

Black beans. Also called turtle beans and *frijoles negros*. Medium-size, oval-shaped beans with an earthy, woodsy flavor, black beans are prevalent in Latin America, the Caribbean, Brazil, Mexico and South and Central America. They are available dried and canned in most grocery stores, and they take 1 to 1½ hours to cook.

Black-eyed peas. Also called black-eyed beans, black-eyed Suzies and cow peas. Medium-sized, light brown, roundish beans with a dark "eye" on their ridges, black-eyed peas are savory, earthy and smooth-flavored. They are available dried, canned and frozen in most supermarkets. They take 45 to 60 minutes to cook.

Chick-peas. Also called garbanzo beans and ceci beans, chick-peas are medium to large in size with a bulging acorn shape and tiny peak. The tan beans have a chewy texture and nutty taste. They are used in the Mediterranean, India, the Caribbean and the Middle East and are available dried and canned in most supermarkets. They take one to two hours to cook.

Cranberry beans. Also called roman beans, shell beans, and tongues of fire. Small- to medium-size with a speckled cranberry-colored skin, these beans turn solid pink when cooked. They are similar to pinto beans in flavor. They are used in Italy and South America and in Native American cooking and are available dried and fresh (in seasonal markets). They take about 45 minutes to cook.

Lentils. There are a myriad of lentils—brown, green, red, yellow and so on. Lentils have a narrow oval shape similar to a thin disk. They are prevalent in Indian, Middle Eastern, North African and European cooking. Dried brown lentils are widely available. Red, green and yellow lentils can be found in Indian

The Basics of Bean Cookery

Like homemade bread, beans gradually come to life, but they need coaxing and an occasional helping hand. Here's how to prepare them.

1. Spread the beans out in a shallow bowl, sort through them and pick out any loose pebbles or sand. Inspect the beans with your fingers and shake the dish as though you were panning for gold.

2. Rinse the beans in cold water.

3. The beans are now ready to be soaked. In addition to rehydration, soaking the beans partially removes the complex sugars that cause indigestion and gas.

Beans will double or triple in size, so soak them in a large pot. One cup of dried beans yields two to three cups of cooked beans.

If time does not permit an overnight soaking, soak the beans at least four hours. Soaking reduces the cooking time and softens the beans.

4. At the end of the soaking time, drain the liquid.

and Asian markets and specialty food stores. They take about 45 minutes to cook.

Lima beans (large). Also called *habas grandes, gigandes,* Burma and Rangoon. Wide beans with a creamy white color and smooth, starchy flavor (similar to small limas), large lima beans take about 1½ hours to cook. They are available both dried and canned in most supermarkets.

Lima beans (small). Also called butter beans and baby limas. Actually the smaller cousin of the large lima, not a younger version, this thumbnail-shaped pale white bean has its roots in South America as well as Africa and Central America. They take about one hour to cook. They are available dried and canned in most supermarkets.

If you are short on time, use the quick-soak method: Place the sorted beans and water in a saucepan and bring to a rolling boil. Simmer for two minutes, then remove from the heat. Allow the beans to sit for one to two hours. Discard the soaking water and then proceed with the cooking process.

One caveat to the quick-soak method: The beans are often not as plump, and they require a longer cooking time. In addition, fewer complex sugars are removed during the process.

5. Combine the beans with three to four times their volume of fresh water in a saucepan and simmer over low heat. Do not cover the pan. Add more hot water if necessary. Cook until the beans are tender or for the recommended cooking time printed on the package.

To check the degree of doneness, remove a few beans from the pot with a slotted spoon and place on a flat surface. Press a fork or spoon against a bean; it should mash easily.

Navy beans. Also called Yankee beans. These are small, oval-shaped white beans that take their name from their prominent role in the U.S. Navy's meal plan. When recipes call for small white beans, they often mean this bean. They are available dried and canned in most supermarkets and take 1 to 1½ hours to cook. This is the bean of Boston baked bean fame and Senate navy bean soup.

Pink beans. Also called pinquito beans. Oval-shaped, smaller than a kidney bean with a pale rose color, these are interchangeable with small red chili beans and pinto beans. They are available dried and canned in most grocery stores and take about one hour to cook.

Pinto beans. These mottled, pinkish brown, oval-shaped beans are rich and full-flavored. When cooked, the faint markings fade to pink. Native to the Americas, pinto beans are a staple of Mexican, Tex-Mex and Southwestern cooking. They are available dried and canned everywhere and take about one hour to cook. This is the bean of choice for refried beans.

Red chili beans. Also called Mexican chili beans and *habas pequeñas coloradas*. Small red beans with a deep burgundy color and oval shape, these are available dried and canned in most supermarkets. They take 1 to 1½ hours to cook. Red chili beans are an acceptable substitute for black beans.

Red kidney beans. Also called Mexican beans, these beans are rich, full-flavored beans with dark and light red hues. They are available dried and canned everywhere and take 1 to 1½ hours to cook. This is the preferred bean for chili.

Split peas. Also called field peas. Split peas are green and yellow whole peas that are halved. When cooked, they lose their shape and meld together. They have a rustic, grassy flavor and are prevalent in Mediterranean, European, Indian and early American cooking. Available everywhere. Great for soups and porridge, they can sometimes be substituted for lentils.

White cannellini beans. Also called white kidney beans. These beans have a smooth texture and slightly nutty flavor. Popular in European cooking, especially Italian, they are available dried and canned in most supermarkets. They take 1 to 1½ hours to cook. These make a good "white" chili and stew.

Lean Bean Recipes

Ready to fall in love with legumes? Try these tasty recipes. To lower the fat content of these dishes even further, use low-fat products where possible instead of the full-fat version.

BRAZILIAN VEGETARIAN FEIJOADA WITH BLACK BEANS

൚

Feijoada (pronounced "fay-ZHWA-duh") is the Brazilian national dish. To retain its distinctive smoky quality without adding meat, use a smidgen of liquid smoke, a prominent ingredient in commercial barbecue sauces.

  1 cup black beans, soaked and drained
  2 tablespoons vegetable oil
  1 large onion, chopped
  1 large red bell pepper, seeded and diced
  1 large tomato, cored and diced
  4 cloves garlic, minced
  1 small jalapeño pepper, seeded and minced
     (wear plastic gloves when handling)
  1 tablespoon rice vinegar or red wine vinegar
1½ teaspoons ground cumin
  1 tablespoon fresh thyme leaves
     or 1 teaspoon dried
  1 teaspoon salt
 ½ teaspoon ground black pepper
 ½ teaspoon liquid smoke
  2 tablespoons minced fresh parsley
4–6 cups cooked white rice

In a large pot, place the beans in plenty of water to cover and cook for 1 hour, until tender. Drain, reserving 1¼ cups of the cooking liquid, and set aside.

Heat the oil in a large saucepan and add the onions and

red peppers. Sauté for about 5 minutes. Add the tomatoes, garlic and jalapeño peppers and cook for 4 minutes more.

Add the beans, reserved cooking liquid, vinegar, cumin, thyme, salt, black pepper and liquid smoke and cook for 30 to 40 minutes over medium heat, stirring occasionally. The mixture should be thick and chunky.

Ladle the *feijoada* into large bowls and sprinkle with parsley. Serve with the rice.

MAKES 6 SERVINGS

 Nutritional Information

Per serving: 483 calories, 7 g. fat (13% of calories), 0 mg. cholesterol, 453 mg. sodium, 7 g. dietary fiber, 15 g. protein, 90 g. carbohydrate.

Two-Bean, Two-Cheese Lasagna with Leafy Green Vegetables

Beans are a natural in this savory, cheesy lasagna filled with leafy greens and herbal seasonings.

- 2 tablespoons olive oil
- 1 medium onion, finely chopped
- 4 cloves garlic, minced
- 1 can (28 ounces) tomato puree
- 2 tomatoes, cored and diced
- 1 cup cooked or canned pink or red beans, drained
- 2 tablespoons dried oregano
- 1 tablespoon dried basil
- 1 teaspoon ground black pepper
- ½ teaspoon salt
- 12–14 uncooked lasagna noodles
- 2–3 cups ricotta cheese
- 2 cups cooked or canned navy beans or other small white beans, drained

1 egg, beaten
2 cups finely chopped mustard greens, spinach or Swiss chard
2 tablespoons minced fresh parsley
2½–3 cups shredded mozzarella cheese

Heat the oil in a medium saucepan, then add the onions and garlic. Cook for 5 to 7 minutes over medium heat. Add the tomato puree, diced tomatoes, pink or red beans, oregano, basil, pepper and salt and cook for 30 minutes, stirring occasionally.

To parboil the lasagna noodles, place 7 or 8 noodles at a time into boiling water to cover and cook for 4 to 6 minutes. Stir occasionally to keep the noodles from sticking together. Remove with a slotted spoon and rinse in cold water. Place the lasagna strips in a single layer on wax paper. Repeat with the remaining noodles.

Preheat the oven to 375°.

In a mixing bowl, combine the ricotta, navy or white beans, eggs, greens and parsley.

Spread a little of the sauce in the bottom of a 9″ × 13″ pan. Cover with a third of the noodles, then half of the ricotta-bean mixture. Spread a third of the remaining sauce over the mixture, sprinkle half of the mozzarella over it, then cover with half of the remaining noodles. Repeat the layering process with half of the remaining sauce, the remaining ricotta mixture and the remaining noodles. Finish with the remaining sauce on top, then sprinkle with the remaining mozzarella.

Bake for 30 to 40 minutes. Let cool for 10 minutes before serving. Cut into rectangles and serve with Italian bread.

MAKES 12 SERVINGS

 ## Nutritional Information

Per serving: 474 calories, 17 g. fat (32% of calories), 70 mg. cholesterol, 555 mg. sodium, 6 g. dietary fiber, 25 g. protein, 56 g. carbohydrate.

Feasts from the East

Sample the Healthiest Traditions of the Orient

VISIT MOST ANY ASIAN COUNTRY for the first time, and what will strike you is the bustling, hectic pace of the people. Workers fill the streets in the day; shops and restaurants stay open late into the night. Food stands are everywhere, and people seem constantly to be either eating snacks or preparing food for sale. Handsome, exotic fruits and vegetables, heaps of greens and cabbages, immense daikon radishes and roots of taro fill infinite stands. Bananas are prepared 20 ways; small rounds of sticky rice studded with black beans are laid out for your inspection on vast banana leaves; vendors stir-fry wondrous concoctions of noodles and vegetables. What strikes you even more is that what seems to be a constantly grazing populace is composed of lean, vital people.

Fascinating recent studies show that Chinese people seem to eat more calories than we do in the West. Yet their cholesterol levels are lower and they weigh less. Incidence of heart disease and breast and colorectal cancers that are extensive in western societies is markedly lower, particularly in rural Asian societies.

The Chinese diet, like other Asian cuisines, focuses on foods from plants—rice and noodles, vegetables and soy products. Meat is expensive where land is more important for cultivating rice than for grazing cattle. Fish, however, can be subcropped in flooded rice paddies, and twice as much fish is consumed in the Orient as anywhere else.

The Chinese eat only one-tenth of the animal protein that

Americans ingest, and their diet contains three times the dietary fiber. Equally important, the average Chinese person gets about 14.5 percent of his calories from fat; the average American gets about 40 percent.

Cornell University research has found that Japanese women, who eat traditionally low-fat diets with a preponderance of tofu as their protein, report fewer hot flashes during

Cooking Rice, Asian-Style

To prepare rice in the Chinese manner: Use short-grain rice, which will yield a more glutinous, clumping rice than long-grain—perfect for eating with chopsticks. Two cups of rice and two cups of water makes six cups of cooked rice.

• Wash the rice, then gently rake it with your fingers. Drain well.

• Place in a pot with measured water and cover.

• Bring to a boil over high heat and immediately stir once to loosen any grains stuck to the bottom.

• Cover, reduce the heat to low and keep covered for about 18 minutes, at which point all the water should be absorbed.

To cook Thai jasmine rice: Jasmine rice, available in most Oriental grocery stores, smells like jasmine flowers and, when cooked, has just a hint of stickiness. Try it with Chinese, Vietnamese, Thai and Indonesian meals.

• Do not rinse the rice.

• In a saucepan, combine 2 cups jasmine rice with 2¾ cups water. Makes 6 cups cooked rice.

• Bring to a boil, cover the pan and reduce to the barest simmer. Cook for 15 to 20 minutes.

menopause and a significantly lower rate of breast cancer than the general female population in the United States.

But take Asian people away from their traditional modes of eating, place them in sedentary jobs and allow them to become westernized, and the risks for cancer and heart disease increase.

So what can an Oriental diet and lifestyle hold for occidental strivers after health? For one thing, without heavy quantities of meat to digest, without a wealth of cream and butter, the body feels light and unweighted soon after a meal based on the carbohydrate cornerstone of rice or noodles. And the greatest benefit by far is the reversal of food proportions. An Asian eats only small portions of meats or stir-fries, using the prepared dishes bite by bite as condiments for the huge amounts of rice he consumes.

A Glossary of Asian Foods

Here are just a few of the most common Asian ingredients that you can use in creative ways to flavor any number of dishes without adding fat or excessive amounts of calories.

Chilies. Hot peppers, red or green, are used whole in Indonesia or shredded and added to curries and soups. Dried pods are added to soups or ground to powders. The Chinese steep them to make a hot flavoring oil.

Cilantro. Also called Chinese parsley or coriander, whole leaves float in Thai soups; handfuls of leaves and stalks are added to Vietnamese *pho*. Use as a side garnish along with cucumber slices to cut hotness of foods.

Fish sauce. This is a strong, pungent seasoning used especially in Thailand (where it's called *nampla*) and Vietnam (where it's called *nuoc mam*). An acquired taste, fish sauce is fermented, looks like soy sauce and is salty to the taste.

Ginger. This is uniformly used in Asian foods. Peel and grate, slice or shred fresh ginger rather than using powdered form. Darker ginger is more intense in flavor but more fibrous than lighter specimens.

Kaffir lime leaves. Used fresh or dry in soups, curries and condiments, kaffir leaves are added like bay leaves to release flavor during cooking. They're good with fish and are available powdered or sometimes fresh in Oriental produce stores.

Lemon grass. This fragrant grass is common in the tropics of Southeast Asia. Slice or mince the compact bulb or add leaves to stews and let them release flavor. Often combined with shrimp paste and turmeric in Thailand and Malaysia, it can also be brewed into tea.

Step-by-Step Stir-Frying

Use a seasoned wok or a large, no-stick frying pan. Cut all ingredients into bite-size pieces; slice meat into long shreds. You can blanch firm vegetables to speed cooking.

Heat the wok over high heat until it starts to smoke. Pour a tablespoon of oil around the pan's middle and cook meat or fish first, in batches. Or coat the wok with a vegetable cooking spray before placing it over heat.

Do not overcrowd the pan; the temperature will drop too low to sear the food. Add chicken stock or orange juice if the pan is dry and food is scorching. Remove cooked food with a slotted spoon and set aside.

Vegetables go in next. Stir-fry scallions, mushrooms, ginger and garlic. Add blanched vegetables. When all are sizzling, return the meat or fish to pan. If following a recipe, add the sauce and cornstarch mixture and turn ingredients rapidly until the sauce becomes glossy. Remember, it's easier to thin than thicken, so add enough cornstarch. You can always toss in a bit of water or stock to thin. If you're not using a sauce, drizzle a little marinade sauce or a low-sodium soy sauce and add spices to your taste.

Shrimp paste. This is a strongly odored paste made from pulverized, salted dried shrimp. It's used in Thailand, Vietnam and Burma. Store covered in oil in a jar. Stir-frying turns acrid flavor to rich seasoning. An acquired taste, perhaps.

Soy sauce. Made from fermented soybeans mixed with wheat, barley or rice, Chinese soy sauce is salty; Japanese soy sauce is slightly sweeter. It comes in light (used particularly with seafoods) or dark versions. Dark has less salt than light. Low-sodium soy sauce is an even healthier alternative, however.

Star anise. With its intense licorice flavor, these eight-pointed seed pods are essential ground in five-spice powder. Put whole pods in stews. (Remove them before serving.) The Thai add one to most simmered dishes.

Tamarind. Sweet, tart, rich paste made from tamarind pods, tamarind is brewed into a delicious cold drink in Thailand and India. Add it to curries and braised dishes. It's a frequent ingredient in Indonesian marinades.

Turmeric. A relative of ginger, this yellow-fleshed root is dried and ground into a slightly bitter, earthy spice. It's essential in curry powder, and the spice by itself is often used with vegetables such as cauliflower. Indonesian cooks combine it with shrimp paste, lemon grass and chili and simmer fish in the mixture.

Mexican Fiesta
Low-Fat South-of-the-Border Favorites

NACHOS OOZING WITH cheese and sour cream. Cheesy quesadillas and enchiladas. Sweet, creamy flan. Why does Mexican food have to be so fattening?

Don't fret—indulge! We've cooked up the following tasty recipes that are low-fat, easy to prepare and spiced just right.

FIESTA DIP

This dip pairs perfectly with pita wedges, low-fat crackers or raw vegetables.

½ cup shredded cucumbers

1 cup nonfat sour cream

½ cup minced sweet red peppers

1 clove garlic, minced

½ teaspoon snipped fresh cilantro

Squeeze excess moisture from the cucumbers; place in a small bowl. Stir in the sour cream, peppers, garlic and cilantro. Chill until needed.

MAKES ABOUT 1½ CUPS

 ## Nutritional Information

Per 2 tablespoons: 14 calories, 0.1 g. fat (1% of calories), 0 mg. cholesterol, 13 mg. sodium, 0.1 g. dietary fiber.

CRISPY TORTILLA CHIPS

Fed up with bagged chips? Keep some tortillas around and crisp up your own treats. Fat and effort are pleasantly low.

12 soft corn tortillas

Cut each tortilla into quarters, then cut each quarter into wedges, sized as you please.

Place the tortilla wedges on a baking sheet and bake at 400° until crisp but not brown, about 5 minutes. Serve with your favorite dip.

MAKES 4 SERVINGS

 ## Nutritional Information

Per serving: 168 calories, 1.8 g. fat (9% of calories), 0 mg. cholesterol, 120 mg. sodium, 0 g. dietary fiber.

TACO BEANS

This healthy, hot and delicious dip is an explosion of flavors.

½ pound lean ground turkey or beef

1 large tomato, seeded and chopped

1 jalapeño pepper, seeded and halved
(wear plastic gloves when handling)

2 scallions, chopped

1 cup cooked pinto beans, mashed

¼ cup diced sweet green peppers

3 tablespoons grated onions

2 cloves garlic, minced

1½ teaspoons chili powder

½ teaspoon ground cumin

¼ cup finely shredded lettuce

¼ cup shredded reduced-fat Cheddar cheese

Crispy Tortilla Chips (see page 273)

Crumble the turkey or beef into a 1½-quart casserole. Microwave on high until the meat is mostly brown, 2 to 3 minutes. Drain off the fat.

While the meat is cooking, combine the tomatoes, jalapeño peppers and scallions in a blender or food processor and process until smooth. Add to the meat. Stir in the beans, green peppers, onions, garlic, chili powder and cumin.

Cover the casserole with a lid, wax paper or vented plastic wrap and microwave on high until hot and bubbly, about 5 minutes.

Top with the lettuce and Cheddar. Serve with the chips.

MAKES 10 SERVINGS

 Nutritional Information

Per serving: 82 calories, 1.4 g. fat (15% of calories), 1 mg. cholesterol, 52 mg. sodium, 0.5 g. dietary fiber.

CRUNCHY LENTIL SALAD

Ready-to-use salsa makes this salad fast and spicy. The jicama, a Mexican root vegetable, adds a nutty flavor.

    2 teaspoons olive oil
    ½ cup chopped red onions
    2 stalks celery, chopped
    2 cloves garlic, minced
    1 cup salsa
    2 tablespoons lime juice
    1 teaspoon horseradish
    ½ teaspoon cumin
    ¾ cup cooked lentils
    ¾ cup cooked corn
    ½ cup chopped jicama
    2 tablespoons snipped fresh flat-leaf parsley

In a large no-stick frying pan over medium heat, warm the oil. Add the onions, celery and garlic; cook, stirring frequently, for 2 minutes. Stir in the salsa, lime juice, horseradish and cumin; simmer the mixture for 2 minutes.

In a medium bowl, pour the salsa dressing over the lentils. Add the corn, jicama and parsley; gently toss to mix well. Serve warm or chilled.

MAKES 4 SERVINGS

 Nutritional Information

Per serving: 259 calories, 4.3 g. fat (14% of calories), 0 mg. cholesterol, 263 mg. sodium, 7.1 g. dietary fiber.

Spinach-and-Cheese Quesadillas

∽

It's time to skip the fat-fry and bake up these healthy, full-flavored quesadillas instead.

½ cup canned chick-peas, rinsed and drained

2 cloves garlic, minced

1 tablespoon water

4 large flour or corn tortillas

1 teaspoon canola oil

½ cup frozen chopped spinach, thawed and squeezed dry

¼ cup chopped roasted sweet red peppers

¼ cup shredded low-fat Cheddar cheese

¼ teaspoon chili powder

Coat a baking sheet with no-stick spray.

In a small food processor, process the chick-peas, garlic and water until smooth. (Or place the ingredients in a bowl and mash well.)

Brush one side of each tortilla with a little of the oil. Place 2 tortillas, oiled side down, on the prepared baking sheet. Spread the tortillas evenly with the bean puree to within ½ inch of their edges. Sprinkle with the spinach, peppers, Cheddar and chili powder.

Top with the remaining 2 tortillas, oiled side up.

Bake at 350° until golden, 10 to 12 minutes. Let cool for at least 5 minutes. Cut each quesadilla into 4 wedges.

Variations: Substitute reduced-fat Monterey Jack cheese for the Cheddar and use corn oil instead of the canola. Top with snipped fresh cilantro. You can easily double this recipe to serve 4.

MAKES 2 SERVINGS

 Nutritional Information

Per serving: 332 calories, 9.6 g. fat (21% of calories), 7 mg. cholesterol, 312 mg. sodium, 5.6 g. dietary fiber.

Turkey Tostadas

Here's a quick and easy one-dish meal with a tasty guacamole accent.

1 pound ground turkey breast

2 cups tomato sauce

½ cup finely chopped onions

¼ cup diced green chili peppers
(wear plastic gloves when handling)

1 teaspoon ground cumin

1 teaspoon chili powder

1 large avocado, peeled and pitted, pit reserved

1 tablespoon lime juice

1 clove garlic, minced

½ teaspoon snipped fresh cilantro (optional)

4 large corn tortillas

½ head iceberg lettuce, shredded

2 medium tomatoes, chopped

¾ cup shredded reduced-fat Cheddar cheese

1 cup low-fat salsa

½ cup nonfat sour cream

Place the turkey in a 2-quart microwave-safe casserole and microwave on high for 2 to 3 minutes. Break up the turkey clumps and microwave on high until the turkey is no longer pink, 1 to 2 minutes. Drain off any fat.

Stir in the tomato sauce, onions, peppers, cumin and chili powder. Microwave on high for 4 to 5 minutes. Set aside.

To make the guacamole, in a medium bowl, mash the avocado with a fork. Stir in the lime juice, garlic and cilantro (if using). Place the avocado pit in the guacamole to keep the color bright, then set the mixture aside. (Remove the pit before serving.)

Place the tortillas on individual plates. Top each with one-quarter of the turkey mixture. Sprinkle each with lettuce, tomatoes and Cheddar. Top each with some of the salsa, sour cream and guacamole.

Variations: For chicken tostadas, replace the turkey with chicken, the cilantro with parsley and the Cheddar with reduced-fat Monterey Jack cheese. Divide or multiply this recipe to serve 2 or 8.

MAKES 4 SERVINGS

 Nutritional Information

> Per serving: 433 calories, 8.9 g. fat (18% of calories), 10 mg. cholesterol, 369 mg. sodium, 10.6 g. dietary fiber.

BEAN-AND-PEPPER ENCHILADAS

For an updated version of a traditional Mexican favorite, try these low-fat, high-fiber enchiladas.

    1 can (16 ounces) pinto beans, rinsed and drained
    1 cup nonfat or part-skim ricotta cheese
  ½ teaspoon chili powder
    1 cup shredded low-fat Cheddar cheese
    1 tablespoon olive oil
    1 cup chopped scallions
    2 cloves garlic, minced
    1 cup chunky salsa
  ¼ cup tomato paste
    1 jalapeño pepper, seeded and finely chopped
       (wear plastic gloves when handling)
  ¼ cup snipped fresh cilantro
    1 tablespoon red wine vinegar
  12 flour tortillas

Coat two 9″ × 13″ baking dishes with no-stick spray; set aside.

Mix the beans, ricotta, chili powder and ¾ cup of the Cheddar in a large bowl. Set aside.

In a large no-stick frying pan over medium heat, warm the oil. Add the scallions and garlic; cook, stirring frequently, until tender, 2 to 3 minutes. Stir in the salsa, tomato paste, peppers and cilantro; bring to a boil. Reduce the heat to low and simmer until the sauce thickens slightly, 5 to 10 minutes. Stir in the vinegar.

Briefly dip a tortilla into the sauce to coat and soften. Place 2 rounded tablespoons of the bean filling on the tortilla. Fold the tortilla to enclose the filling, then place, seam side down, in one of the baking dishes. Repeat with the remaining tortillas.

Spoon the remaining sauce evenly over the enchiladas. Sprinkle with the remaining ¼ cup Cheddar.

Cover the baking dishes loosely with foil and bake the enchiladas at 350° until the cheese has melted and the sauce is hot and bubbly, 15 to 20 minutes.

MAKES 6 SERVINGS

 Nutritional Information

Per serving: 401 calories, 11.4 g. fat (25% of calories), 83.6 mg. cholesterol, 175 mg. sodium, 6.3 g. dietary fiber.

HONEY-VANILLA POACHED PEARS

No fiesta is complete without a memorable sweet treat based on a Mexican-inspired flan.

6 pears

3 tablespoons vanilla

3 tablespoons honey

3 cups Honey-Vanilla Custard (see opposite page)

Peel the pears; cut them in half and place them in a Dutch oven. Cover the pears with water.

In a small bowl, combine the vanilla and honey; add to the water for poaching the pears. Bring the sweetened water to a boil; reduce the heat, cover and simmer until the pears are just tender but not soft, about 15 minutes. Remove the pears from the water with a slotted spoon, place in a dish and refrigerate.

To serve, place 2 pear halves in each of 6 dessert bowls; spoon about ½ cup custard over each portion.

Variation: Replace the custard with vanilla nonfat yogurt or frozen yogurt.

MAKES 6 SERVINGS

 Nutritional Information

Per serving: 287 calories, 4.2 g. fat (13% of calories), 9 mg. cholesterol, 81 mg. sodium, 4.4 g. dietary fiber.

Honey-Vanilla Custard

*Creamy, sweet flan is the traditional Mexican meal-ender. This
version is as guiltless as it is good-tasting.*

    3 cups evaporated skim milk
    3 tablespoons cornstarch
    ½ cup honey
    ½ cup fat-free egg substitute
    1½ teaspoons vanilla
    1 tablespoon reconstituted butter-flavored mix

In a medium saucepan, combine the milk, cornstarch
and honey; mix well. Cook over low heat, stirring constantly,
until the mixture combines and thickens. Be careful not to
boil or scorch. Remove from the heat.

In a small bowl, stir about ¼ cup of the warm honey-
milk mixture into the egg substitute; return the mixture with
the eggs to the honey-milk mixture in the saucepan. Place over
low heat (do not boil) and cook, stirring constantly, until the
custard is thick, smooth and creamy, about 15 minutes.

Stir in the vanilla. Add the butter-flavored mix and continue stirring until blended. Transfer to a casserole and cover
with plastic wrap. Chill for at least 2 hours.

MAKES 6 SERVINGS

 Nutritional Information

Per serving (approximately 1 cup each): 141 calories, 2.3 g. fat (15% of
calories), 9 mg. cholesterol, 118 mg. sodium, 0.1 g. dietary fiber.

....

Simple Salmon

Succulent Fish That Is a Snap to Prepare

FLASHING THROUGH THE COLD, dark streams of Scotland, surging up the coast of Oregon and Washington, gliding majestically through the waters of Alaska, sleek, silvery salmon never fail to excite fishermen. And whether it's set out poached and garnished as the decorative center of attention at a banquet table, laden smoked and savory on a bagel or barbecued and striped from the grill, the beautiful peachy pink flesh of salmon never fails to excite the most discriminating of eaters.

Salmon, our most adaptable, most kingly fish, is surging in popularity these days, not only for its versatility and wonderful taste but also for its wondrous nutritional benefits.

Time was when an expensive cut of red meat used to be the dish of choice at party banquet tables. But salmon is no longer just a dish fit for kings or expense-account diners. With salmon being farmed in greater quantities than ever, the prices for these exquisite fish and the quality available are better than at any time in history.

The extraordinary thing about salmon is that it remains unique, distinctively itself, no matter how it's cooked. Salmon done up in Cajun or Chinese or Catalan style always seems to taste of salmon alone rather than its attempted style.

Other fish may disappear into generic "fishiness" under a deluge of frying or saucing, but salmon always stands up for itself.

The reasons that we also should stand up for salmon are legion. Salmon is, without a doubt, the most palatable and delicate of all the fish that are considered oily. Nutritionists are the first to point out that the oily fish contain omega-3 fatty acids, one of the "good" kinds of fat. Omega-3 fatty acids are associated with reduced risk of heart attacks and strokes and with less risk of inflammatory diseases such as rheumatoid arthritis.

Salmon, like all fish, is super-low in artery-clogging saturated fat. Plus it stocks some vitamin A, vitamin D, B vitamins and potassium. For an extra dose of calcium, crumble the bones in canned salmon and eat them, too.

Get It while It's Fresh

When shopping for fresh salmon, here are some tips for selecting the freshest fish.

• Use your nose, eyes and fingers when you select your purchase. Bring fish up to your nose and sniff for a slightly salty, fresh seaweed odor, as opposed to a strong, oily odor.

• Feel the flesh of the fish. There should be a firm, slightly elastic quality—a certain resistance to the flesh. If you are buying a whole fish or side, run a finger over the scales. They should stick tightly to the salmon's skin. Press the fish with your finger—if it leaves an indentation, it's probably old fish. Cut fillets and steaks should feel firm, not watery and not flaccid.

• If you don't want to deal with pinbones, purchase tail sections of salmon, which are always boneless. (The best way to remove pinbones from salmon, by the way, is with a pair of pliers.)

Here's an easy way to judge the quality of canned salmon. Stand the can upright for a night at room temperature. Then open the can, gently depress the fish and spoon off some of the oil that comes to the surface. The more oil and the richer the color, the better the quality of the fish. The fish should also feel firm and be an attractive pink color.

Storing and Cooking Salmon

Purchase only as much fresh salmon as you want to cook in the next 24 hours. Put it on a bed of ice in a flat container in the coldest part of the refrigerator as soon as possible after its purchase. Cover with wax paper. If you're lucky enough to have a fisherman in the family, freshly caught salmon can be frozen in a deep freezer chest—never in the freezer section of your refrigerator. (It's not cold enough to freeze the fish quickly.)

Thaw frozen salmon for no more than 30 minutes at room temperature. It should be partially defrosted but still firm.

Be particularly conscious of cooking times and simplicity of preparation when you cook salmon. Measure salmon fillets and steaks at their thickest points, then apply the ten-minute rule in all cooking situations, from poaching to boiling: For each inch of thickness at the fish's thickest point, allow ten minutes of cooking. Baste with water once or twice if you're broiling or baking. Cook the flesh until it's opaque, then test the fish by gently inserting a fork or knife point at the thickest section of the fish, gently pulling the fish aside. Look for flaking with no raw center.

If you are cooking the fish in a sauced preparation or wrapping it in foil with a stuffing in the cavity, add an extra 5 minutes to the cooking time.

And if you ever have the opportunity to cook a very large, freshly caught Alaskan king salmon, consider preparing the fish in the native Eskimo way: During the laying of the Alaskan pipeline, workers frequently came back to their work camps to a dinner of freshly caught salmon that had been cleaned, slit open, stuffed with carrots and onions, then wrapped and slowly baked under a bed of coals throughout the afternoon to a succulent melting goodness.

Whether you choose to broil a salmon steak or poach a tail section, whether you make salmon cakes or salmon burgers from canned fish, there are certain accompaniments that seem to attend salmon with special grace.

Yes, salmon goes well with either white, wild or brown

rice. But don't forget that staple Russian dish *kulebiaka*, in which salmon is baked along with mushrooms and a garnish of hard-cooked eggs in a bed of cracked bulgur wheat or buckwheat kasha. Salmon can stand up to these healthy grains with no loss of flavor.

There is no prettier salmon presentation then a blue and white plate, a serving of pink fish and a green vegetable. A quick sauté of spinach and garlic, fresh steamed asparagus or broccoli all do nicely. But for wonderful counterpoint delicacy, try the crunch of cucumbers. Sliced cucumbers become wonderful crisp salad when simply dressed with yogurt, lemons and fresh chopped dill. Cooked cucumbers are wonderful also. Peel and carve them into seedless ovals, then simply parboil them until crisp-tender; dress them with fresh dill and a few drops of olive oil.

One of the freshest ways to serve salmon is in the *lomi lomi* style of Hawaii. Cube cooked or lightly smoked salmon and mix it with equal amounts of cubed tomatoes, mild red onions and minced parsley. Dress it with lemon juice and a few drops of olive oil and mound it on a bed of lettuce leaves for an island-style presentation.

··

Heart and Soy
Discover the Health Benefits of Soy Foods

IMAGINE LOWERING YOUR RISK of breast and other cancers, heart disease and osteoporosis simply by making minor modifications to the way you prepare many of the foods you already eat—and maybe adding a few new recipes. Or lessening—even eliminating—menopause symptoms. That's what can happen when you add soy foods to your daily diet. Foods made from soybeans are some of the most versatile and
(continued on page 288)

SWEET POPPY DRESSING

ᔥ

2 tablespoons Dijon-style mustard
2 tablespoons honey
  juice of 1 lemon
1 cup light plain soy milk
2 teaspoons poppy seeds
½ teaspoon paprika
¼ teaspoon grated orange rind

In a bowl, mix the mustard and honey. Then add the lemon juice, milk, poppy seeds, paprika and orange rind; mix well. Drizzle on green salad or serve as vegetable dip.

BANANA PANCAKES

ᔥ

3 tablespoons soy oil
1¼ cups plain soy milk
1¾ teaspoons baking powder
1 teaspoon salt
1 cup whole-wheat flour
½ cup soy flour
2 bananas, thinly sliced

In a bowl, mix the soy oil and milk; blend in the baking powder, salt, whole-wheat flour, soy flour and bananas. Cook on a lightly oiled griddle. Serve with fruit.

TOFU MEATBALLS

1 large onion, sliced

1 cup fresh parsley

1/2 cup egg substitute

2 packages (10 1/2 ounces each) extra-firm low-fat tofu, drained

1/2 cup seasoned bread crumbs

1/2 teaspoon dried basil

1/2 teaspoon oregano

1/2 teaspoon black pepper

1/2 teaspoon dry mustard

1/4 teaspoon fennel seeds

1 clove garlic, crushed

1/4 cup grated Parmesan cheese (can be low-fat)

3 tablespoons tomato sauce

1/4 cup whole-wheat flour

In a food processor or blender, mix the onions, parsley and egg substitute until smooth. Transfer to a bowl. Stir in the tofu, bread crumbs, basil, oregano, pepper, mustard, fennel seeds, garlic, Parmesan and tomato sauce. Form into balls, roll the balls in the flour and then place in a lightly greased baking pan. Bake at 350° for 35 minutes.

delicious products imaginable—and the health benefits of consuming soy food are nothing short of striking.

The King of Beans, the Bean of Kings

Soybeans have a long, rich history in Eastern world cuisine. They were discovered on the windy plains of east Asia centuries ago and, according to Chinese tradition, were named as one of the five sacred crops by emperor Sheng-Nung, who reigned 5,000 years ago.

Soybeans revolutionized the diets of Asian countries, and inventive cooks created numerous soy-based staples that added nutrition and variety to the Asian diet, like soy milk, tofu, tempeh, miso and soy sauce.

Today most of these foods are quickly becoming familiar fare in many American kitchens. What's more, American food companies have expanded the list of authentic soy foods: There's a whole new generation of soy-based products that look and taste like meat and dairy products, such as tofu burgers and soy cheese. During the past decade more than 2,000 new soy products have made their way into food stores. Soy foods are better tasting and more convenient than ever.

While some soy products are fairly high in fat, others are available in light or fat-free versions. So check labels carefully in order to purchase the foods that best help meet your nutritional objectives. Still, the fats in soy foods are unsaturated and therefore less damaging than the saturated fats found in animal foods such as beef, pork, chicken, fish and dairy products.

An All-Natural "Disease Shield"

Soybeans pack a lot of nutrition. The high protein quality of soy is comparable to meat and eggs. In fact, the U.S. government recognizes soy as a protein alternative equivalent to meat. What's more, soybeans and soy foods are rich in iron, B vitamins, calcium and zinc and are cholesterol-free, very low in saturated fat and free of lactose (milk sugar).

Studies show that replacing animal protein in the diet

with soy protein, or simply adding soy protein to the diet, significantly reduces blood cholesterol levels, even in people already on low-fat, low-cholesterol diets.

Studies show that people who consume soy foods on a regular basis are less likely to develop cancer than those who rarely consume these foods. Scientists are especially excited about a component of soybeans called genistein. Genistein is a powerful anticarcinogen. In test tubes it directly inhibits the growth of a wide range of cancer cells. To derive the potential benefits of genistein, it is necessary to eat soy foods; no other commonly consumed food contains it.

Cooking with Soy: Simply Delicious

Adding soy to your diet can be as simple as pouring a cup of soy milk over your morning cereal. The versatility of soy foods makes them easy to incorporate into many of your favorite dishes. Here's a listing of the most popular soy foods and how to use them.

Soybeans. These grow in fuzzy green pods, usually two round beans to a pod, on bushy, hip-high plants. They lose their green color as they mature and ripen into hard, dry beans. Most soybeans are yellow, although brown and black varieties are available as well. To cook mature soybeans, soak them in water for several hours, then simmer for two to three hours until soft. Cooked soybeans should be soft enough to crush easily between your tongue and the roof of your mouth. They have a deep, nutty flavor that stands up well in spicy chili sauces or flavorful stews or soups.

Soy flour. This can boost the protein content of baked goods as well as give them a dose of cholesterol-lowering soy protein. Replace one-quarter to one-half of the flour in muffins, cakes, cookies, pancakes and quick breads with soy flour. For yeast-raised breads, use about one-quarter soy flour. Soy flour is free of gluten, so yeast-raised breads made with it are slightly more dense. But these breads also have a wonderful nutty flavor and moist texture.

Soy flour also can be used to replace eggs in baking. Replace each egg with one tablespoon soy flour and two table-spoons water.

Texturized soy protein (TSP). This is a high-protein, fat-free, dehydrated soy product. While TSP doesn't sound overly appetizing, many people have found it a tasty meat substitute. Rehydrated TSP has a texture similar to ground beef and can be used in tacos, meat loaf, chili, spaghetti sauce or any dish normally prepared with ground beef or ground turkey. Substitute TSP for half of the meat or use TSP alone. Store TSP in an airtight container for several months. Once it is rehydrated, TSP must be refrigerated and should be used within four days.

Soy milk. A rich, creamy liquid expressed from cooked and soaked soybeans, this lactose-free beverage can be used in nearly any way that whole milk can, from baked goods to creamy puddings and soups to frosty shakes. It also tastes great plain.

Soy milk is usually sold in aseptic packages. Once the package is opened, soy milk should be refrigerated and used within a week. Soy milk comes in a variety of flavors including plain, chocolate, almond, vanilla and carob.

Tofu. Made by curdling soy milk, in much the way that cheese is made from whole milk, tofu has the consistency of a soft cheese. There are several varieties of tofu, from extra-firm tofu to "silken," which has the creamy texture of a delicate custard. Tofu is usually sold in the produce section of grocery stores.

Tofu soaks up the flavors of the ingredients with which it is cooked, so it's right at home in a pot of the spiciest chili and in the creamiest cheesecake. Tofu also makes wonderful dips—just use it in place of sour cream. Crumble firm tofu into stews and soups, use it to replace part of the meat in a meat loaf or sauté it with your favorite spices and serve in a pita pocket. Tofu also can be frozen. Try basting defrosted tofu with a tangy barbecue sauce and cooking it on the grill.

Tempeh (pronounced TEM-pay). This is made by combining cooked soybeans and grains with a fermenting culture. The result is a chunky cake of beans with a chewy texture and a rich, smoky flavor. It's a wonderful meat substitute: The flavor of tempeh particularly lends itself to spicy dishes such as tacos and chili. Tempeh is also delicious grilled and adapts well to barbecue sauce or sweet-and-sour sauces. Tempeh is available in natural food stores and specialty markets in the freezer or refrigerator case. Frozen tempeh will keep for several months. Defrosted tempeh can be refrigerated for up to a week.

Meat analogs. These products made from soy and other ingredients look and taste like meat; try them in sandwiches, stews, soups, even on the grill. Look for soy-based hot dogs, deli meats, sausages and burgers in natural food stores and in supermarkets.

You'll also find a growing number of dairy analogs—soy products with the look and taste of cheese and ice cream.

Miso. A paste with the consistency of peanut butter, miso is made from soybeans, grain, salt and a beneficial bacteria culture. The mixture is aged for a year or more. Miso can be used in place of salt or soy sauce. It's also used to make broth for soup: Just dissolve a quarter-cup in a quart of water. Keep it tightly covered and store it in the refrigerator. Miso is available in natural food stores or in Asian markets.

Are You a Part-Time Vegetarian?

A record 5 percent of the population—over 12 million Americans—now say no to animal foods. And millions of others can be classified as quasi-vegetarians. These people typically eat chicken and fish a few times a week and steak rarely, if at all. Like vegetarians, quasi-vegetarians' meatless meals center around items such as salads, pasta, vegetables, whole grains, legumes—and oftentimes, soy foods.

Study after study confirms that the less meat you eat, the healthier you are likely to be. For women that translates into extra protection against breast cancer, unpleasant menopause symptoms and osteoporosis as well as heart disease and cancer.

Note: Avoid miso if you're on a sodium-restricted diet.

Soy oil. The most commonly consumed oil in the United States, soy oil contains omega-3 fatty acids, a type of fat found primarily in fish oils that may provide a number of important health benefits. Like all vegetable oils, soy oil is cholesterol-free and is also low in saturated fatty acids. Soy oil is tasteless, so use it in recipes in which you want the flavor of other ingredients to shine through.

The Ripe Stuff
A Fresh Look at Fresh Fruit

LUSCIOUS BERRIES PILED HIGH in pretty goblets . . . plates of sliced peaches, kiwifruit and melons arranged in still-life perfection . . . scoops of elegant fruit ices accented with sprigs of mint or basil. Fruit is lovely to look at, sweet on the tongue and one of nature's nutritional powerhouses.

For good health, nutritionists tell us, we should aim to eat two to four servings of fruit each day. Fruit's packed with soluble fiber, which keeps our cholesterol levels in check, insoluble fiber, which keeps our digestion on track, and a host of vitamins, minerals and other important nutrients.

Selecting fruit at its peak usually requires more than a pinch or a poke, but it's easier than you might think. That goes for serving it, too. Fresh, ripe fruit can be savored out of hand or served simply with other foods that complement them. Here's *Prevention* magazine's guide to choosing and serving the earth's sweetest bounty.

Berries

Low in calories and brimming with fiber, berries are a dieter's dream dessert. Select berries by checking the bottom of their box for staining; bruised or overripe berries spoil quickly. Sniff the box—if there's no aroma, there will be no taste, either.

Blackberries. Of all the summer fruits, blackberries get the highest rating for fiber. One cup has as much total fiber as one cup of cooked oat bran.

The blacker the berries, the riper and sweeter they will be. Rinse blackberries before using. So fragile and intense are these berries that they are best served fresh and adorned simply— with a dollop of vanilla nonfat yogurt, for example.

Blueberries. Ripe berries should feel firm and look dark blue with a silvery blush. Fresh blueberries can be stored up to five days. Rinse the berries just before serving, picking out loose stems or leaves and discarding soft or bruised berries. This fruit takes wonderfully to mixed-fruit compotes, tarts and cobblers.

Raspberries. Another star of fiber and flavor, raspberries are very perishable. Buy these berries the same day you intend to eat them. Choose and use raspberries just like blackberries. Or for an elegant dessert, pour sparkling apple juice over ripe raspberries.

Strawberries. One cup of these berries deliver more than 100 percent of the Daily Value (DV) of vitamin C and pack more fiber than two slices of whole-wheat bread. Ripe strawberries should be bright red with unwilted caps. Select berries with the least amount of yellow and avoid those with white shoulders. Rinse strawberries just before hulling. You can serve these berries in mild balsamic vinegar, an Italian favorite.

Melons

Low in calories (50 to 60 calories per cup), melons are among the most refreshing summer fruits. Melons don't ripen once they have left the vine, so avoid underripe melons. One ripeness test: Press gently on the blossom end; the melon should give slightly. To maximize the flavor of most melons, let them sit for a day or two at room temperature. They won't grow any sweeter, but they will become softer and juicier.

Serve at room temperature or refrigerate no more than an hour or so, except for watermelon, which tastes best very cold.

Cantaloupe. One cup of cantaloupe cubes also delivers more than 100 percent of the DV for vitamin C and has more potassium than a banana. This is the melon richest in beta-carotene, too. Cantaloupe should have a pronounced indentation at the stem end—called a full slip—which indicates that the fruit was ripe enough to slip off the vine. Sniff the stem end of room-temperature cantaloupes for fragrance. Without a whiff of sweetness, the melon will have no flavor.

Honeydew. Give honeydew the sniff test, as you would cantaloupe. The rind of a ripe honeydew is creamy yellow and coated with a slightly sticky film, like tiny droplets of honey. Large melons make the best eating, since they grow closest to the root of the plant and are meatier. Those with smooth, markedly greenish rinds will not ripen, so avoid them.

Honeydew tastes wonderful doused with lime juice or drizzled with a few drops of raspberry vinegar and a sprinkling of cilantro.

Watermelon. Choose watermelon with bright-green stems, which signals that they came from a live vine. The underside of a ripe watermelon's rind should look yellowish, while the rest may be a deep green. Thumping a watermelon isn't the best way to test ripeness; the only foolproof way is to buy a cut one. Once cut open, those melons with the most deeply colored flesh and the darkest seeds are the ripest. Avoid melons with a hard, white streak running lengthwise through the melon. If the watermelon's flesh is cracked and grainy, it's too ripe.

For a festive-looking dessert, toss chunks or balls of watermelon, honeydew, cantaloupe and pineapple with a splash of lime or pineapple juice. Add sherbet or fruit ice scooped with a melon baller and serve in a scooped-out melon half.

Stone Fruits

Apricots. Test apricots for ripeness—as you should most stone fruits—by pressing them gently between your palms.

A Trio of Icy Treats

Try whipping up one or more of these fresh fruit ices. It's easy. Put the fruit in a blender and blend until smooth. Then pour into a bowl or shallow pan and place in the freezer. Stir every 15 minutes or so to break up ice crystals and prevent the mixture from freezing solid too fast. These take at least 1½ to 2 hours—and six to eight vigorous stirrings—to finish. Don't prepare them more than 8 hours in advance; ices are best served right from the freezer. If you must work ahead, cover the finished product tightly with foil to prevent flavor loss. Serve in chilled dishes, garnished with mint leaves or fresh fruit sections.

Try the following flavor combinations. Each recipe serves two.

FENNEL-HONEYDEW ICE

1 cup honeydew puree
¼ teaspoon fennel seed
¼ teaspoon lime juice

BERRY ICE

1 cup berry puree (use raspberries, blueberries or strawberries)
⅓ cup water
1 tablespoon honey
½ teaspoon lemon juice

NUTMEG-PEACH ICE

1 peach, sliced
3 tablespoons nonfat yogurt
   dash grated nutmeg

(Pinching them will bruise the fruit.) Apricots should yield to gentle pressure and emit a slight perfume. Choose the rosiest apricots and avoid hard fruits that shade to yellow-green. Set on a counter away from heat or direct sunlight or store in a paper bag at room temperature until very soft, then use immediately. Don't wash them until just before serving.

Poach apricots in honey-flavored syrup and top with nonfat yogurt. Or serve them up fresh with yogurt, a sprinkling of cinnamon and a spoonful of honey.

Mangoes. A cup of mango chunks delivers even more beta-carotene than a cup of cantaloupe and is an especially rich source of soluble fiber. Some people compare the mango's flavor to a medley of apricot and melon; others, to a cross between peaches and pineapple. An occasional whiff of a turpentine-like smell signals underripeness, while ripe fruit give off a sweet aroma. Choose mangoes that have a warm-tinged blush and that give slightly when you press them between your palms. Store them at cool room temperature, since heat can affect their flavor.

Serve mango slices plain with a squeeze of lemon or lime juice or over nonfat frozen yogurt. Or puree mango chunks in a food processor and use as a sauce over other fruits, rice pudding or angel food cake.

Nectarines. Select bright, plump fruit and avoid hard, dull fruit or fruit that looks a bit shriveled. Press a nectarine along its seam; if it is ripe, it will yield to gentle pressure there. You may have to leave firm nectarines on a kitchen counter for a day or two to soften or put them in a paper bag with an apple or a banana to speed ripening. Coat their flesh lightly with lemon juice to prevent darkening once they are sliced and exposed to air.

Try stuffing nectarines with minced ginger, chopped almonds and a drizzle of maple syrup. Bake for 20 minutes at 350°, then cool and serve with nonfat yogurt.

Peaches. Don't pinch peaches to feel the slight give of the skin that signals ripening. Instead, look at the color of the stem end. Choose only those fruits that show no green tint. Sniff them for perfume; scent signals ripeness better than color, since a peach's blush is determined by its variety, not by its maturity. See "Nectarines" for softening instructions and a simple serving idea.

Plums. Plums rank among the high scorers in delivering cholesterol-lowering soluble fiber. Choose plums that are brightly colored and slightly soft at the stem and tip; avoid plums with wrinkled, mottled or cracked skin. Pick plums from the top of a grocer's pile where they have not been bruised by the weight of the fruit above them. To ripen plums, place them in a loosely closed paper bag and leave at room temperature. Then refrigerate them if you won't be eating them immediately.

Plums can be baked or pureed and flavored with lemon juice, almond extract and spices. You can also bake plums in Brown Betty or cobbler-style.

Sweet cherries. Select plump, shiny, deep-colored fruit with fresh green stems. Handle cherries with care. Keep them refrigerated and avoid exposing them to sunlight or water until you are ready to eat them. Bings, with mahogany skin and

Throw a Peach on the Barbie

Grilled fruits complement any summer barbecue. Stone fruits, such as apricots, nectarines, peaches and plums, can be halved, pitted and grilled, cut side down, to start. Mangoes can be cut into ½-inch-thick slices. Turn once to finish cooking. Depending on how hot your grill is, cook no more than three to five minutes on each side. While most berries are too small to grill, strawberries can be skewered and combined with other fruits. Cherries can be pitted and skewered as well. Skewered fruits should take no longer than one to two minutes on each side. Lightly drizzle grilled fruits with honey or sprinkle them lightly with finely chopped nuts and cinnamon. Or simply serve warm off the grill with nonfat frozen yogurt.

sweet flesh, are particularly good stewed in just a bit of water, honey, cinnamon and a scrape of nutmeg. Stew briefly, then puree and use the delicious sauce to coat sliced pears.

Figs. Fresh figs offer a wealth of fiber, especially the soluble kind. Look for plump figs that are rich in color and soft to the touch. While figs are easily bruised, you should pick them up (gingerly) by their bodies rather than their stems, which detach all too easily when the fruits are mature. In the Mediterranean region, fig trees are planted among almond, walnut, citrus, olive and grape crops, and all of these foods marry well with figs.

For a classic French presentation, serve fresh figs on a bed of crushed ice in a handsome dish. Puree and strain fresh raspberries and let each person pour the sauce over her own serving. Or peel the rind of an orange in long strips. Simmer in honey and water until the strips are candied. Pour over room-temperature figs and serve.

Kiwifruit. Ounce for ounce, kiwis contain even more vitamin C than oranges and are a leading source of soluble fiber. The kiwi's taste has been described as a cross between a banana and a strawberry, with a touch of tartness. A ripe kiwi's texture is almost custardlike. Choose fruit that yield to pressure with a slight give. The brownish green skin is edible if you briskly rub off the prickly fuzz with a dish towel. Or peel the fruit and slice it crosswise so you can see the sunburst of small black seeds in the center of its bright green flesh.

Drizzle kiwi slices with a touch of honey or coat them with raspberry puree.

Credits

"Carpal Tunnel Syndrome: A Nutritional Twist for a Painful Wrist" on page 85, "Jet Lag: Don't Let Air Travel Drag You Down" on page 159 and "Pancreatitis: Eat to Beat a Belly-ache" on page 177 were adapted from *Doctor, What Should I Eat?* by Isadore Rosenfeld, M.D. Copyright © 1994 by Isadore Rosenfeld, M.D. Reprinted by permission of Random House, Inc.

"Depression: Eat to Feel Better, Not Blue" on page 100 was adapted from *Food and Mood* by Elizabeth Somer, M.A. R.D. Copyright © 1995 by Elizabeth Somer. Reprinted by permission of Henry Holt and Co., Inc.

"The Tasty Bean: Going Meatless Can Be Marvelous" on page 260 was adapted from the book *Lean Bean Cuisine*, copyright © 1995 by Jay Solomon, Prima Publishing, Rocklin, Calif. Reprinted by permission.

"Honey-Vanilla Poached Pears" on page 280 and "Honey-Vanilla Custard" on page 281 by Paulette Mitchell originally appeared in *Quick and Healthy Cooking*. Copyright © 1995 by Paulette Mitchell. Reprinted by permission.

"Crispy Tortilla Chips" on page 273, "Taco Beans" on page 274 and "Turkey Tostadas" on page 277 by Sharon Claessens originally appeared in *Quick and Healthy Cooking*. Copyright © 1995 by Sharon Claessens. Reprinted by permission.

"Heart and Soy: Discover the Health Benefits of Soy Foods" on page 285 was adapted from "Super-Charge Your Diet with Soy Foods!" originally published in *Women's Health Letter* in March 1995. Copyright © 1995 by *Women's Health Letter*. Reprinted by permission.

Index

Note: <u>Underscored</u> page references indicate boxed text.